AF228878

CLIMATE CHANGE IMPACT
Human Health

Andrea C. Nakaya

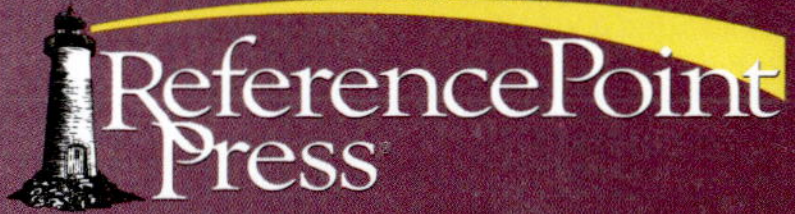

ReferencePoint Press®

San Diego, CA

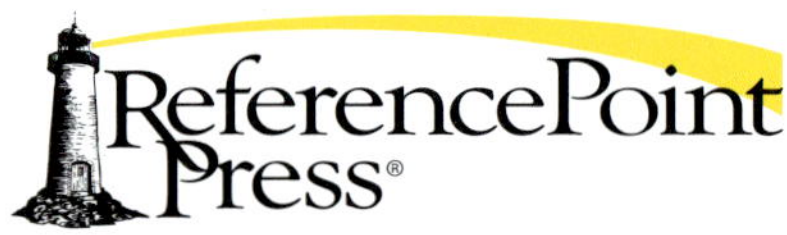

About the Author

Andrea C. Nakaya, a native of New Zealand, holds a BA in English and an MA in communications from San Diego State University. She has written and edited numerous articles and more than fifty books on current issues. She currently lives in Eagle, Idaho, with her husband and their two children.

For more information, contact:
ReferencePoint Press, Inc.
PO Box 27779
San Diego, CA 92198
www.ReferencePointPress.com

LIBRARY OF CONGRESS CATALOGING-IN-PUBLICATION DATA

Names: Nakaya, Andrea C., 1976- author.
Title: Climate change impact : human health / by Andrea C. Nakaya.
Other titles: Human health
Description: San Diego, CA : ReferencePoint Press, Inc., 2025. | Series: Climate change impact | Includes bibliographical references and index.
Identifiers: LCCN 2024009913 (print) | LCCN 2024009914 (ebook) | ISBN 9781678208288 (library binding) | ISBN 9781678208295 (ebook)
Subjects: LCSH: Climatic changes--Health aspects. | Climatic changes--Health aspects--Juvenile literature. | Health--Juvenile literature.
Classification: LCC RA793 .N35 2025 (print) | LCC RA793 (ebook) | DDC 613/.1--dc23/eng/20240319
LC record available at https://lccn.loc.gov/2024009913
LC ebook record available at https://lccn.loc.gov/2024009914

CONTENTS

Health and Climate Are Inseparable

The year 2023 was one of climate records. According to the National Oceanic and Atmospheric Administration, that year saw the hottest worldwide August since the agency began keeping climate records 174 years ago. Ocean temperatures also reached record highs, and Antarctic sea ice was at a record low. In addition, as reported by the *New York Times*, there were twenty-three weather and climate disasters in the United States, causing more than $1 billion in damages each—another record. All of these records demonstrate that the earth's climate is changing. As it does, people's lives are being affected in many ways. One of the most important impacts that climate change is having is on human health.

This is because human health is closely linked to the climate. The US Environmental Protection Agency (EPA) explains, "Climate change affects the food we eat, the air we breathe, the water we drink, and the places that provide us with shelter."[1] The close ties between the climate and people's most basic needs mean that when the climate changes, so does health. While climate change can have some positive effects on health, experts believe that most of its impacts are disruptive and potentially harmful to society. For instance, the EPA explains that some areas are experiencing more intense storms than usual due to the changing climate, and although there are some potential benefits from these storms, these are generally outweighed by their harms. The EPA says, "While increased precipitation can replenish water supplies and support agriculture, intense storms can damage property, cause loss of life and population displacement, and temporarily disrupt essential services such as transportation, telecommunications, energy, and water supplies."[2] *The Fifth National Climate Assessment*, a US government report on climate change, confirms that the health-related consequences of climate change are likely to be primarily negative. It warns, "Although a few US regions or sectors may experience limited or short-term benefits from climate change, adverse impacts already far outweigh any positive effects and will increasingly eclipse benefits with additional warming."[3]

Serious Consequences

According to the EPA, there are two main ways that the changing climate can negatively affect health. One is that it can make the health problems that people already face more serious and more frequent. An example of this is the fact that warmer weather can increase air pollution, which can worsen breathing problems in people with asthma. The other way climate change can harm health is by creating health problems in people or places where these problems have not existed previously. For example, warming is increasing the range of mosquitoes, resulting in malaria and other mosquito-borne illnesses in regions where they have never occurred before.

The health-related threats from climate change are significant. The world is already experiencing heat waves, degraded air quality, more frequent extreme weather events, growth in disease-causing vectors, and reduced water quality as the climate changes, and these are all having negative impacts on human health. The World Health Organization (WHO) predicts that climate change will cause 250,000 deaths worldwide during 2030 to 2050, and by 2030 it will cause $2 billion to $4 billion yearly in damages to health. The WHO stresses, "Climate change is the single biggest health threat facing humanity."[4] In addition to increased rates of physical illness and death, researchers have recently discovered that worry over climate change is leading to negative mental health effects among a significant number of people.

Something That Will Affect Everyone

Overall, most experts agree that the health-related threats of climate change are substantial and are growing. Warns *The Fifth National Climate Assessment*, "It is an established fact that climate change is harming physical, mental, spiritual, and community health and well-being," and that "climate-related hazards will continue to grow, increasing morbidity and mortality across all regions of the US."[5] The same trend is occurring around the planet.

While everyone will be affected by climate change, certain groups of people are more vulnerable to its effects. The EPA explains, "Climate change does not affect all people equally. Some

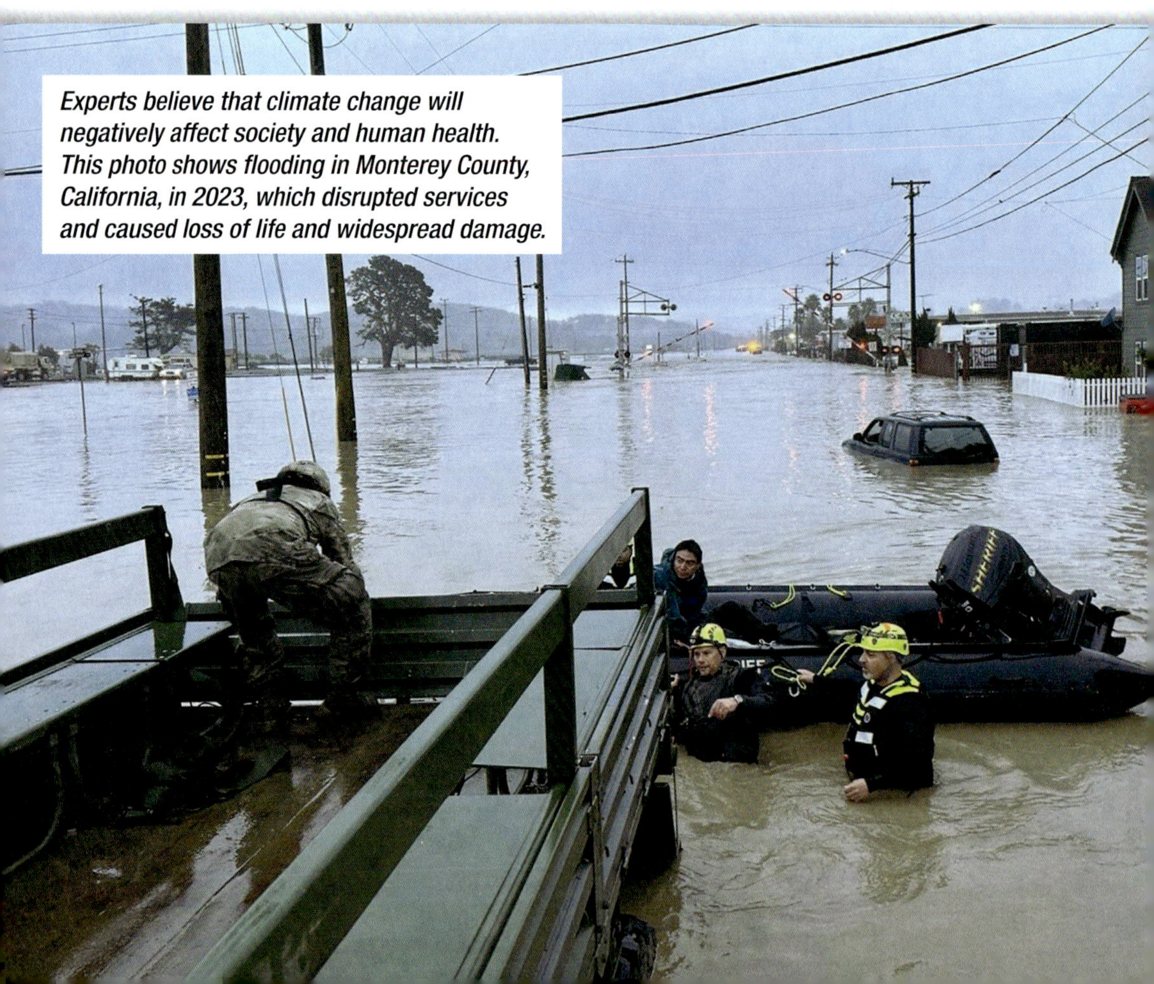

Experts believe that climate change will negatively affect society and human health. This photo shows flooding in Monterey County, California, in 2023, which disrupted services and caused loss of life and widespread damage.

communities experience disproportionate impacts because of existing vulnerabilities, historical patterns of inequity, socioeconomic disparities, and systemic environmental injustices." Unfortunately, adds the agency, "people who already face the greatest burdens are often the ones affected most by climate change."[6]

However, although this threat is real, there are also many ways for humankind to combat it. Everyone can do things to reduce the harms of climate change, including taking actions to reduce future changes to the climate and finding ways to mitigate those changes that have already occurred. These things are happening around the world in ways both big and small. Srilata Kammila, head of climate change adaptation for the United Nations Development Programme, stresses that climate change is tied to the most basic determinants of human health—air, water, food, and shelter—and maintains that it is something that everyone in the world needs to keep working to fix. She says, "This is the most pressing health and humanitarian challenge of the 21st century."[7]

CHAPTER ONE

Heat-Related Threats to Human Health

On November 17, 2023, thousands of excited concertgoers filled a stadium in Rio de Janeiro, Brazil, to see singer Taylor Swift perform. Among them was twenty-three-year-old Ana Clara Benevides Machado. According to a *Washington Post* article, "Pictures showed her . . . smiling and wearing friendship bracelets popularized among Swift fans."[8] However, the weather that day was not ideal for an outdoor concert. While it was only spring, Rio de Janeiro was in the midst of an unusual and record-breaking heat wave. Temperatures were over 100°F (37.8°C), and the heat index, which is a measure of both temperature and humidity, was the highest that had ever been measured there.

Many people struggled to handle the overwhelming heat. One concertgoer says, "It was easily the hottest day in my life, there was no wind and the place was overcrowded. During Taylor's show, I noticed a lot of people getting dizzy from the heat, feeling sick, and friends and family running around the stadium looking for water to hydrate."[9] Machado also started feeling unwell and was taken to paramedics, then transported to the hospital. Soon after, she died. Swift canceled the next night's show, stating, "The safety and well-being of my fans, fellow performers and crew has to and always will come first."[10] A spring heat wave like this is virtually unprecedented in Rio de Janeiro; however, there and in cities all over the world, extreme heat is becoming more and more common because of climate change. Machado's death is just one example of how heat-related events are affecting human health.

A Warming Planet

There is ample evidence that the world is becoming hotter and that heat waves are growing in frequency and severity. *The Fifth National Climate Assessment* reports that the United States now experiences more numerous and longer periods of dangerous heat than in the past. It says, "Across 50 large US cities, the US Global Change Research Program heat wave indicator . . . shows that the average number of heat waves has doubled since the 1980s, and the length of the heat wave season has increased from about 40 days to about 70 days."[11]

The United States is not the only country where heat waves are becoming more commonplace. World Weather Attribution, an organization that studies the way climate change is affecting weather, found that while extreme heat waves were once unusual worldwide, that is no longer the case. It says, "These events are not rare anymore today. North America, Europe and China have experienced heat waves increasingly frequently over the last years as a result of warming caused by human activities, hence the current heat waves are not rare in today's climate."[12]

Heat Can Be Deadly

Extreme and prolonged heat can cause serious health problems and can even be deadly. In a recent study on the health effects of extreme heat, researchers explain that the body can deal with extreme heat up to a certain point. They say, "The human body is designed to self-regulate its temperature, even when exposed to severe cold or heat. The body adapts to extreme heat by both

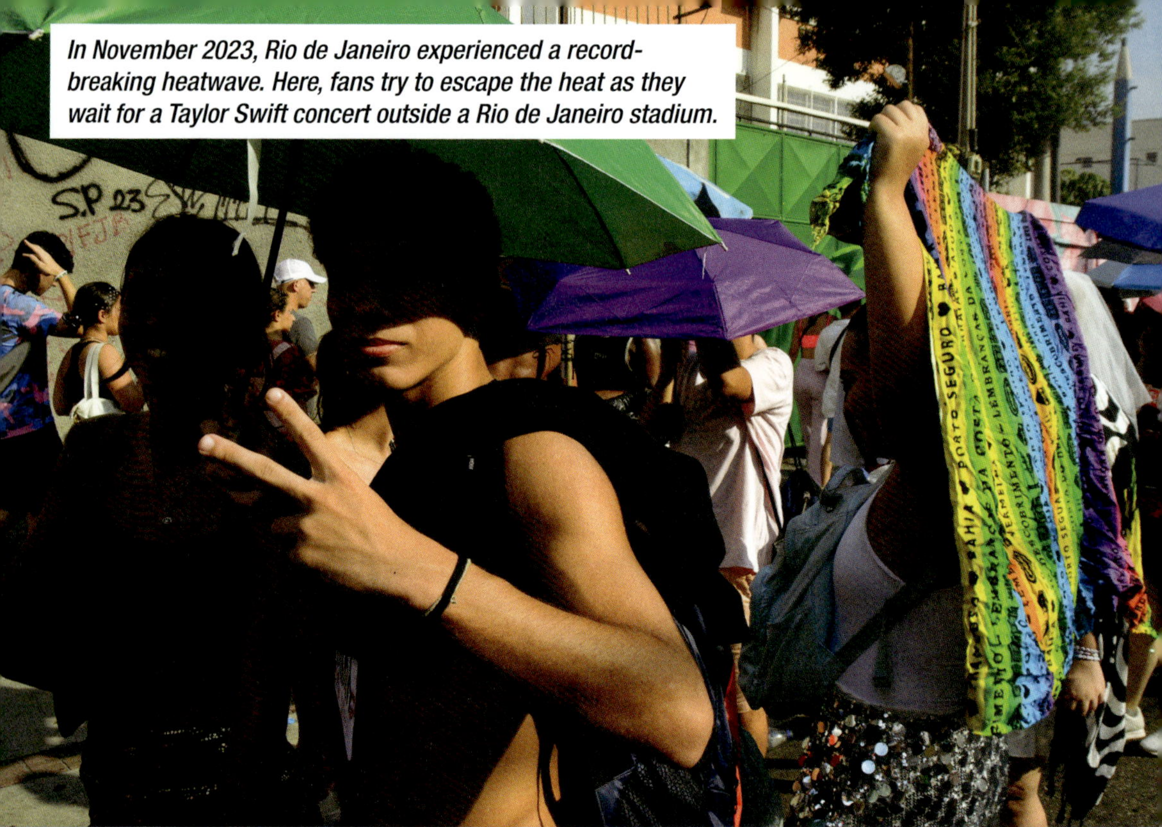

In November 2023, Rio de Janeiro experienced a record-breaking heatwave. Here, fans try to escape the heat as they wait for a Taylor Swift concert outside a Rio de Janeiro stadium.

increasing perspiration (sweating) and evaporative cooling." However, the researchers point out that when the weather gets too hot, this temperature regulation system can stop working. They state, "Natural systems for thermoregulation can fail when the body experiences prolonged heat exposure, when humidity levels interfere with evaporation, and when dehydration and salt depletion reduce blood pressure and cause electrolyte imbalance."[13]

When the body starts to have trouble regulating itself in the heat, people can experience a range of health problems. They might start by getting heat cramps, which are painful muscle cramps and spasms. Heat exhaustion is more severe than heat cramps and happens when the body starts struggling to keep itself from getting too hot and a person loses too much water and salt. The symptoms of heat exhaustion can include cold and clammy skin, a racing heart, nausea, dizziness, tiredness, and a headache. Sabrina describes her experience with heat exhaustion on the National Weather Service website. She says:

I chose to hike alone, without water, and I did not check the weather. It turned out to be a hot day with no breeze. I brought a juice box and told myself I wouldn't need more. When I got thirsty, I melted a handful of snow. When I returned to camp, I was clammy, shaking, ash gray, had a splitting headache, and felt nauseous. I looked and felt awful; the camp nurse said I had heat exhaustion. It took over a day to recover.[14]

The most dangerous type of heat-related illness is heatstroke. This happens when a person's body temperature rises above 103°F (39.4°C). Symptoms can include a rapid pulse, a decrease in perspiration, disorientation, and loss of consciousness. Heatstroke is a medical emergency. Danelle Eby Choate shares her story of heatstroke. She says, "I was mowing my yard (about an acre, on a riding lawn mower) mid morning in August in Tennessee. I was taking 5 minute breaks, sipping water, trying to cool down, but I wanted to finish, so I ignored the lack of sweat and cramping in my arms. After I finished, I took a shower. Got dizzy, passed out, busted my head open."[15] Choate says she had to be taken to a doctor, who used staples to close the cut on her head.

Health Problems Caused by Heat

Exposure to prolonged or extreme heat can cause health problems in addition to heat exhaustion and heatstroke. It can lead to heart disease, result in pregnancy complications, worsen asthma and chronic obstructive pulmonary disease, and give rise to kidney and blood pressure problems. Certain groups of people are more vulnerable to its harm. Young children and the elderly are especially susceptible to heat-related illness because their bodies are less efficient at regulating temperature than those of other age groups. *The Fifth National Climate Assessment* states, "Heat-related health impacts are greatest among children, adults over age 65, those with disabilities, people with mental health or substance-use disorders; and those who are pregnant, lack access to cooling, or engage in outdoor labor and activities."[16] It also finds that Black, Asian, and Latino communities are more likely than others to be harmed by extreme heat, as well as homeless populations, low-income groups, and those who live in urban areas.

Heat can also exacerbate existing health problems. People with medical conditions such as diabetes, heart disease, and respiratory illness are more likely to experience health problems from heat than those who do not suffer from these conditions. In an article in the *Guardian*, the author reports that the majority of heat-related deaths actually occur in this way, explaining, "Only a small share of heat-related deaths come from heatstroke. In most cases, hot weather kills people by stopping the body from coping

Heat Is the Biggest Killer

Many different types of weather can kill, but experts say that heat kills more people every year than any other type of weather event. Leana S. Wen, a *Washington Post* contributing columnist and a professor at George Washington University's Milken Institute School of Public Health, says, "Extreme heat already kills more Americans than hurricanes, floods or any other weather-related emergency." Melissa Guardaro is an extreme-heat researcher at Arizona State University. She points out that many people do not realize just how deadly heat is because, unlike some other types of extreme weather events, it does not leave a visible trail of destruction. She says, "We kind of have a joke here that we show a picture of before a heat wave, and then we show a picture after a heat wave, and it's the same picture. And that's part of the problem, because people see tornadoes and houses are upended and hurricanes and trees and utility poles. [Heat] is this invisible killer."

Leana S. Wen, "Extreme Heat Is Threatening Virtually Every Aspect of Human Health," *Washington Post*, August 1, 2023. www.washingtonpost.com.

Quoted in David Pogue, "Extreme Heat, the Most Lethal Climate Disaster," CBS News, August 6, 2023. www.cbsnews.com.

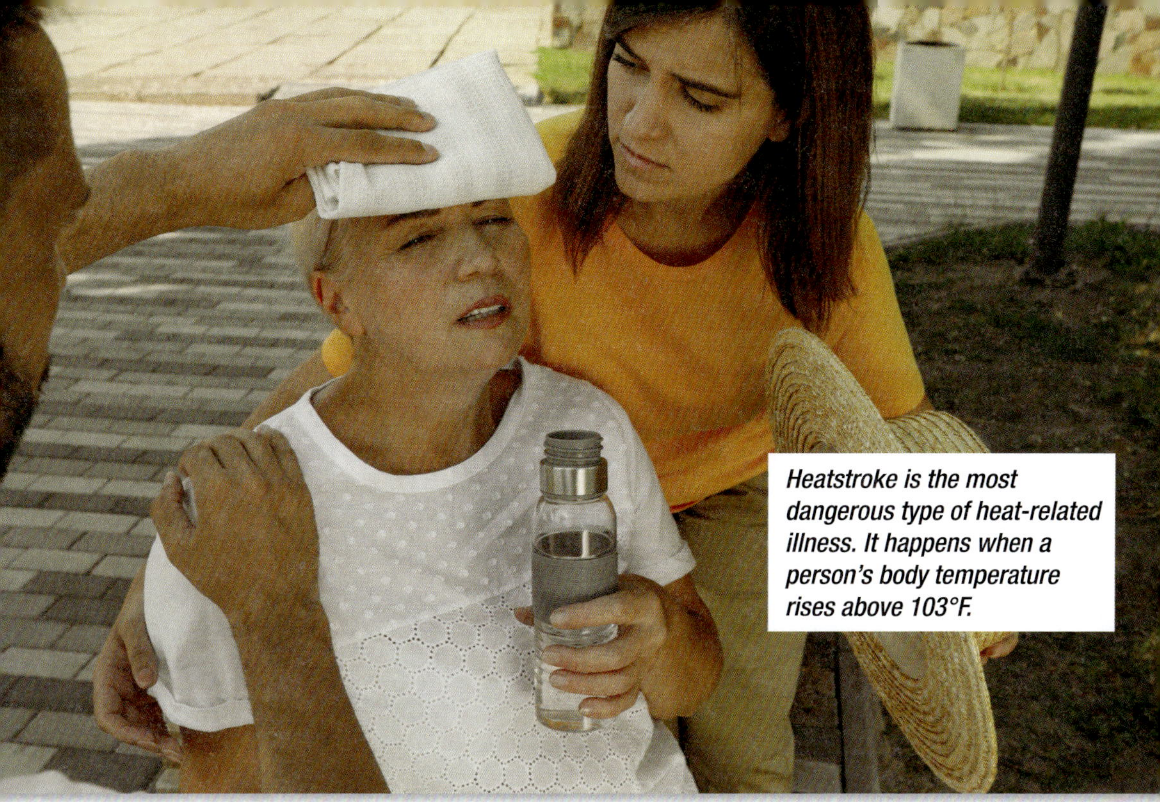

Heatstroke is the most dangerous type of heat-related illness. It happens when a person's body temperature rises above 103°F.

with existing health problems like heart and lung disease."[17] The article quotes Dr. Ángel Abad, who lives in Madrid, Spain, where summer heat waves are common. Abad says that he often sees patients whose existing health problems become worse because of the heat. He says, "It's very frequent in summer in Spain in our hospitals. . . . The patient cannot breathe. The heart starts failing. The [underlying] problem becomes stronger."[18]

One group of researchers analyzed hundreds of studies to understand how extreme heat can affect the health of people who have cardiovascular disease. They looked at studies that examined the effect of high temperatures on cardiovascular disease and discovered that a 1.78°F (1°C) increase in temperature was associated with a significant rise in cardiovascular disease–related death. This finding is significant, because as the researchers explain, "internationally, cardiovascular disease is the leading cause of disease burden, accounting for one-third of all deaths."[19] This means that an increase in cardiovascular disease–related deaths is likely to mean a significant increase in deaths worldwide.

Heat and Outdoor Workers

Some jobs can only be done outdoors. Much of the work that takes place on farms and in construction, for instance, happens outdoors. Even when it gets hot outside, people in these types of jobs are expected to work. This makes them more vulnerable than other workers to heat-related harms. According to a 2021 government report, more than eight hundred US workers died from heat ailments during 1992 to 2017; however, the authors of the report stress that the real number of deaths is likely to be much higher. They say, "This is likely a vast underestimate, given that injuries and illnesses are underreported in the US, especially in the sectors employing vulnerable and often undocumented workers. Further, heat is not always recognized as a cause of heat-induced injuries or deaths and can easily be misclassified, because many of the symptoms overlap with other more common diagnoses." The authors predict that in the future, outdoor workers will face an increasing number of unsafe workdays due to heat.

US Department of Labor, "Heat Illness Prevention in Outdoor and Indoor Work Settings," Reginfo.gov, 2021. www.reginfo.gov.

A Major Health Threat

In recent years extreme heat waves around the world have killed many people. For instance, Europe experienced record-breaking heat waves in both 2022 and 2023. According to a July 2023 report in the journal *Nature*, the 2022 heat waves claimed a staggering number of victims; more than sixty thousand people died. In the United States, Phoenix experienced its longest ever heat wave in 2023, with more than thirty consecutive days when the temperature reached 110°F (43.3°C) or higher. Average lows were about 90°F (32.2°C), which meant that it was very difficult for people to ever cool down. Many hospitals were overwhelmed with patients suffering from dehydration, heatstroke, and other heat-related problems. Patients also included a significant number of people suffering contact burns from hot surfaces. "It doesn't cool down here at all and surface temps can get so ridiculously high and people can get burns in a matter of seconds,"[20] medical center communications director Michael Murphy told CNN. "The heat is taking a major toll," emergency room doctor Frank LoVecchio said. He reported that every time he worked a shift, he saw three to four cases of people who would have died without emergency treatment. He added, "The hospital has not been this busy with overflow since a few peaks in the COVID pandemic."[21] Nearly five hundred people died in the 2023 Phoenix heat wave.

Because many parts of the world do not keep accurate records on heat-related deaths, the extent of the threat posed by heat waves is actually likely to be underestimated. The Virginia Commonwealth University and the Center for American Progress conducted a study in 2022 and 2023 in which they used data from Virginia to get a better understanding of how extreme heat impacts health. They concluded, "The health impact of extreme heat is larger than official statistics suggest. For every person seeking medical attention for heat-related illness, countless more suffer at home, either from heat-related illness or complications from preexisting conditions."[22]

Ways to Stay Cooler

While heat is threatening health around the world, many people have found innovative ways to deal with it. One growing solution is to design buildings that absorb less heat than traditional

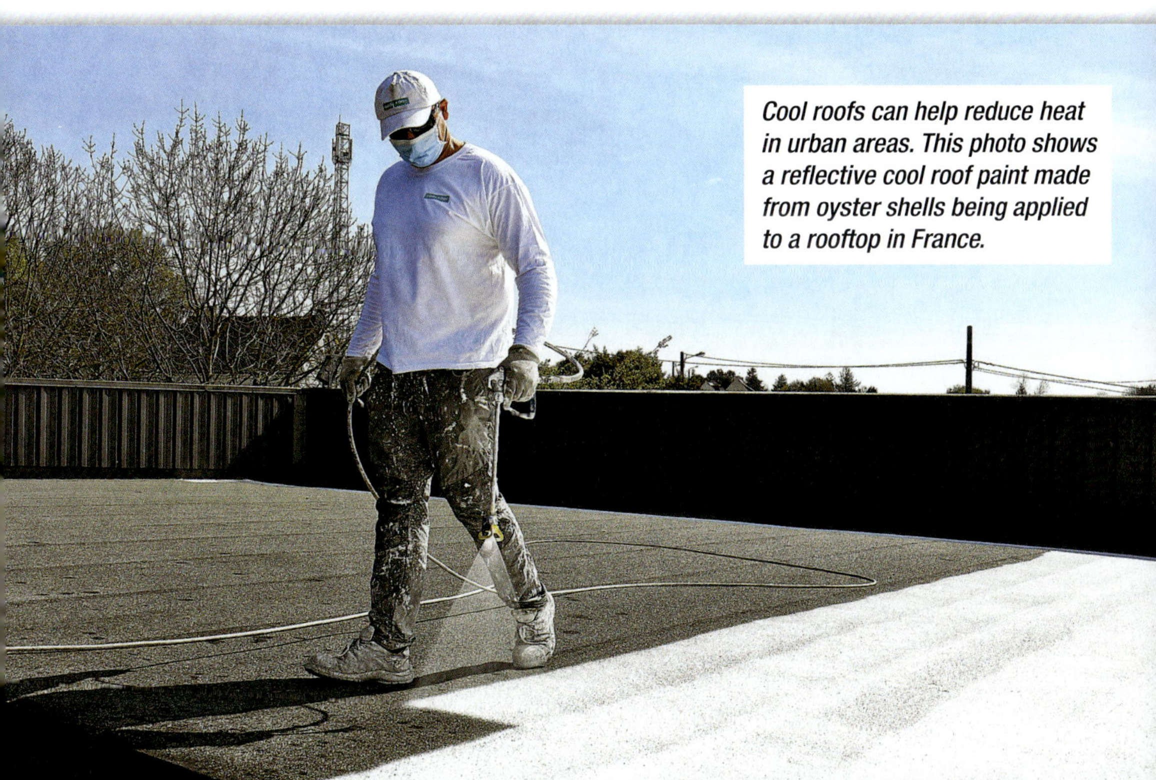

Cool roofs can help reduce heat in urban areas. This photo shows a reflective cool roof paint made from oyster shells being applied to a rooftop in France.

structures when the weather becomes hot. For example, meteorologist Bonnie Schneider describes using what are known as "cool roofs" as a strategy for reducing heat in urban areas. This involves using light-colored coatings or surfaces on roofs, which will reflect heat away from the building. She says that this can be very effective, explaining, "On a typical summer afternoon, a cool-colored roof that reflects 35 percent of the sunlight will stay about 22°F cooler than a traditional roof that looks the same but reflects only 10 percent of the sun."[23]

Another common solution to the warming climate is to increase green spaces, which can also have a significant cooling effect. Cities tend to be much warmer than rural areas because they have a high concentration of surfaces like sidewalks and buildings that absorb heat. This is known as the urban heat island effect. In contrast, trees and other plants create shade, deflect heat, and can substantially reduce the temperature on hot days. Many cities have started to work on expanding their green spaces to combat warming. For instance, the city of Paris has announced that it plans to become one of the greenest cities in Europe. According to one news article, "By 2026, mayor Hidalgo has pledged to plant more than 170,000 trees across the capital, with 50 percent of the city covered by planted areas by 2030. To help make that happen, building codes have been loosened so it is much easier for Parisians to plant trees in their neighbourhoods."[24]

There have also been attempts to increase green spaces in the United States. For example, in 2023 the government released $1 billion to plant trees in cities and towns across the country. Efforts like these are important because heat can be harmful to health in many ways, and most experts believe that humanity's future is very likely to include a planet that is even warmer than it is now.

CHAPTER TWO

How Changing Air Quality Impacts Health

The average adult breathes twelve to twenty times per minute. Children breathe even more frequently. If a person stops breathing, death can occur within minutes. As these facts reveal, air is crucial to human survival. However, the quality of that air is also critically important. When people do not breathe clean air, they can experience health problems, including allergies, asthma, and lung disease. Unfortunately, breathing clean air is already a challenge in many places. For instance, the American Lung Association finds that in the United States, one in three people lives in an area with unhealthy air quality. As climate change alters the quality of the air in many parts of the world, breathing clean air is likely to become an even greater challenge for many people in the future.

Climate Change Is Worsening Air Quality

There is widespread evidence that climate change is worsening air quality by increasing common pollutants. When researchers measure air quality, two of the things they usually look at are ground-level ozone and particulate matter pollution, which are very common types of pollution. Ground-level ozone is a gas that is created from pollutants that come from cars, factories, and other sources and is harmful to human health. Particulate matter consists of tiny

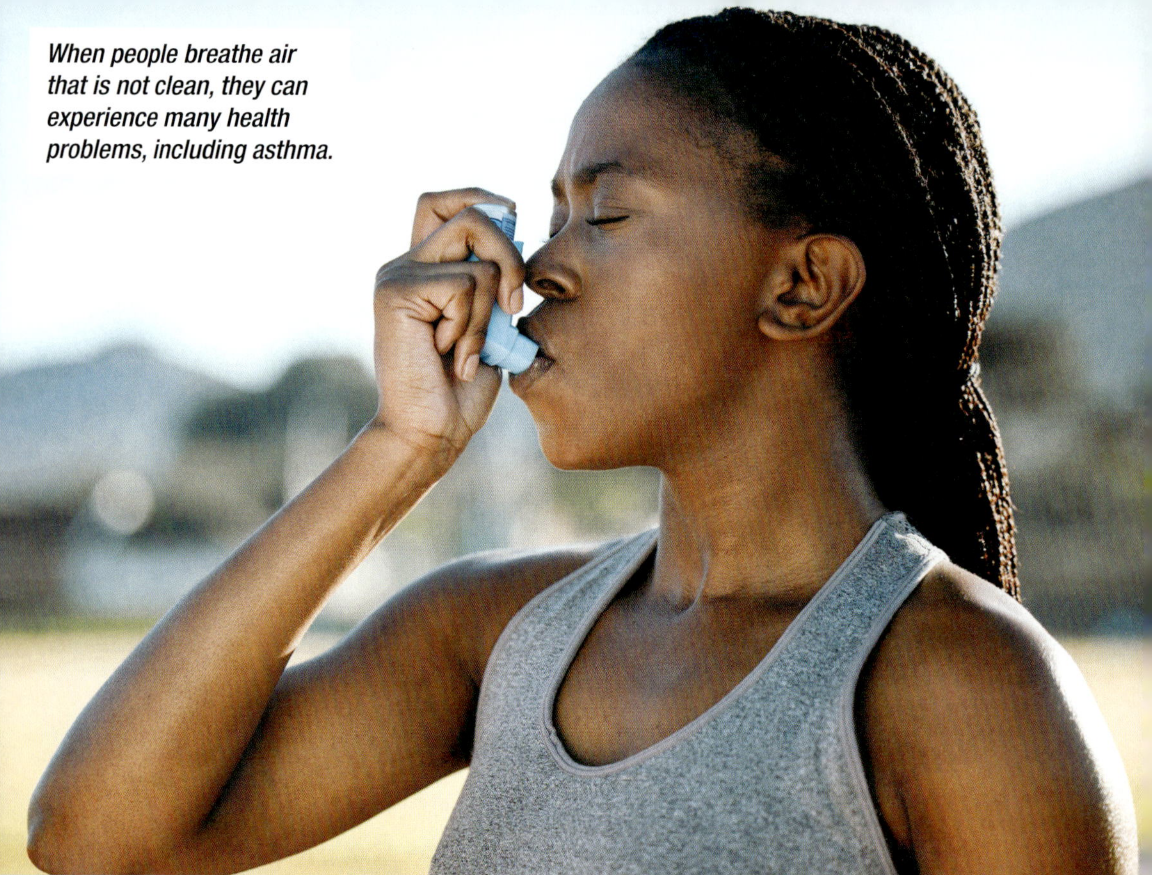

particles of harmful pollutants like soot, metals, ash, and dust. When the weather is warmer, the chemical reactions that create ozone increase, resulting in more ozone pollution. Warming also makes areas of stagnant air and dry, dusty air more likely, both of which can trap and concentrate particulate matter. Research shows that as the climate warms, all of these things are happening and that both ground-level ozone and particulate matter pollution are becoming worse.

The American Lung Association tracks these pollutants in the United States and publishes its findings in a yearly report called "State of the Air." For many years this report showed that the country was making progress in improving its air quality. However, in 2023 the organization found that climate change is stalling that progress in many places, stating, "From the beginning, the findings in 'State of the Air' have reflected the successes of the [1970] Clean Air Act, as emissions from transportation, power plants and manufacturing have been reduced. In recent years, however, the findings of the report have added to the evidence that a changing climate is making it harder to protect human health."[25] The publication goes on to say that within the past three years, almost half a million more people lived in areas that received a rating of F for unhealthy levels of particulate matter, more than in any of the previous ten reports. Similar increases in unhealthy air can be seen in many other parts of the world.

Climate change is also leading to drought conditions in many places and increasing the occurrence of wildfires, making smoke—another type of air pollution—more prevalent. Researchers from Stanford University recently created an artificial intelligence model to track wildfire smoke in the United States so that they could make predictions about future trends. Lead researcher Marissa Childs says, "We found that people are being exposed to more days with wildfire smoke and more extreme days with high levels of fine particulate matter from smoke."[26] The researchers discovered that ten years ago, fewer than half a million people lived in areas that had unhealthy smoke levels for at least one day a year. Now, they explain, that number has increased twenty-seven-fold, to more than 8 million people. Keith Bein, an atmospheric scientist at the University of California, Davis, agrees that it has become much more common for people to be exposed to wildfire smoke. "People were once exposed once or twice in a lifetime," he says. "Now it's happening every summer and for longer."[27]

In addition to intensifying smoke and pollution, climate change is altering air quality by raising pollen levels. The Centers for Disease Control and Prevention (CDC) explains that pollen is a part of the air that people breathe, and the amount of pollen varies throughout the year. The CDC says, "Pollen grains are tiny 'seeds' dispersed from flowering plants, trees, grass, and weeds. The amount and type of pollen in the air depends on the season and geographic region."[28] As a result of climate change, however, the agency explains that carbon dioxide levels have increased, temperatures have warmed, and precipitation patterns have changed—and that these factors are causing higher pollen counts and longer pollen seasons in many places.

Poor Air Quality Harms Human Health

Increases in air pollution, smoke, and pollen all pose a threat to human health. Polluted air can cause problems ranging from short-term irritation to serious long-term conditions. Common health problems caused by air pollution include wheezing and coughing, asthma, lung disease, heart attacks and strokes, metabolic disorders, preterm birth and low birth weight, and cancer. The American Lung Association says, "Years of scientific research have clearly established that particle pollution and ozone are a threat to human health at every stage of life."[29] The WHO calls air pollution "a major environmental threat,"[30] and says that it is one of the main causes of death worldwide, killing about 7 million people each year. The National Weather Service estimates that in the United States, more than one hundred thousand people die yearly as a result of air pollution and that air pollution–related illnesses cost more than $150 billion annually.

Wildfire smoke in particular is known to be bad for human health. In addition to harmful particulate matter that is small enough to get deep into people's lungs and thereby into their bloodstream, wildfire smoke also contains pollutants from whatever is burning. As fires have become more frequent and larger, that often includes not only forests but buildings as well. An article posted by the University of California, San Francisco, explains why that matters. The author states, "Wildfire smoke contains a mix of chemicals, including those released by homes as they burn—from household cleaners to asbestos siding. Depending on what's fueling the fire, wildfire smoke can include things like sulfuric acid, dust and mold."[31] Exercise physiologist and wildfire firefighter Joe Domitrovich has studied the impact of smoke on firefighters. He explains, "Wildland firefighters are spending 100 days each summer fighting these fires."[32] This means that they are exposed to a lot of smoke, and their experiences can reveal something about its health effects. Domitrovich found that retired woodland firefighters, who had spent a lifetime being exposed to wildfire smoke, had a greater-than-normal risk of cardiovascular disease and lung cancer.

Like air pollution, pollen also has a significant impact on human health. Pollen particles in the air can cause an allergic reaction, resulting in sneezing, congestion, a runny nose, and red and itchy eyes. They can also cause or worsen more serious problems such as asthma and other respiratory illnesses. The CDC says, "Medical costs linked with pollen exceed $3 billion every year."[33] Further, people who experience allergic reactions may get tired more easily, find it harder to concentrate, have lower energy levels, and have higher levels of stress and anxiety than people who do not. Theresa MacPhail, a medical anthropologist and author of *Allergic: Our Irritated Bodies in a Changing World*, says that pollen is causing health concerns for ever-greater numbers of people. She explains, "Over the last decade, the number of adults and children diagnosed with mild, moderate, or severe allergies has been steadily increasing worldwide with each passing year. Billions of people worldwide, an estimated 30–40 percent of the general global population, currently have some form of allergic disease."[34]

A Growing Problem

Around the world, it is becoming more common than ever for people to find themselves breathing polluted air and experiencing negative health consequences as a result. For instance, in the summer of 2023, Canada endured a record-breaking fire season that most experts believe would not have occurred without climate change. In total, there were thousands of fires, which burned millions of acres and spread smoke across both Canada and the United States. Millions of people breathed in harmful smoke for days or even weeks. In June, New York City had some of the unhealthiest air in the world.

A CDC study found that this air had a noticeable impact on the health of Americans. Researchers discovered that during the days when there was smoke from the 2023 fires, asthma-related emergency room visits in the United States were 17 percent higher than usual. Canadian fire scientist Mike Flannigan warns that years like this are likely to become relatively routine in the future because warmer weather is causing fire seasons to start earlier and last longer. He says, "We have to learn to live with fire and smoke, that's the new reality."[35]

High levels of pollen are also becoming a growing concern for some people. In many areas pollen counts are significantly higher and pollen seasons last longer than in the past. Neelu Tummala, an ear, nose, and throat specialist, says, "The pollen season

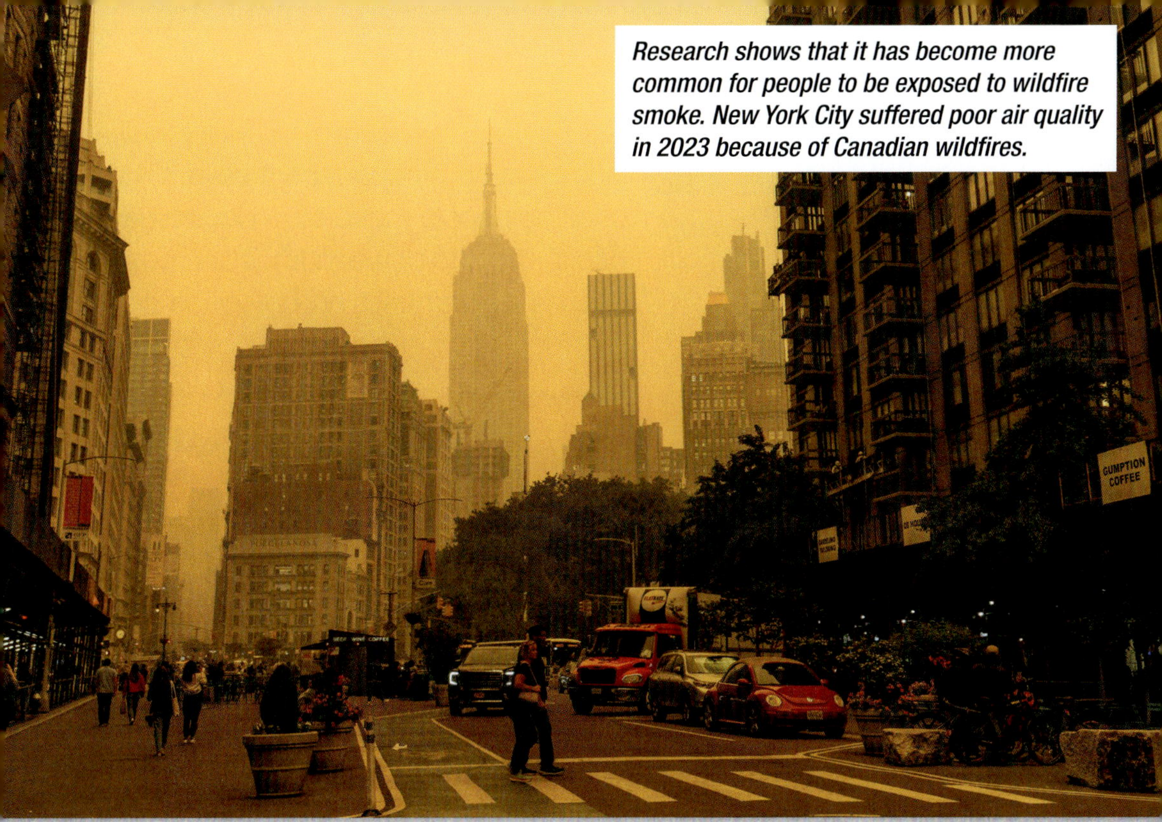

Research shows that it has become more common for people to be exposed to wildfire smoke. New York City suffered poor air quality in 2023 because of Canadian wildfires.

right now is about three weeks longer than it was 30 years ago, and there's about 20% more pollen in the air."[36] These changes mean that some people are finding that their allergies are becoming more severe, while others are developing allergies for the first time. Clifford Bassett is an allergist at NYU Langone Health in New York City. He reports, "What I see is people coming in for the first time, especially over the last five, seven years or so. They will always say, 'I don't understand how this is happening to me.'"[37]

Cleaning Up the Air

While polluted air is a major health threat, many things can be done to lessen the problem. Greenhouse gas emissions are a major cause of air pollution, so reducing emissions is one of the best ways to reduce air pollution. This can be done by large entities like manufacturers, but it is also important at an individual level. Although some people may believe that their own actions are too insignificant to impact emissions, that is far from true. *The Fifth National Climate*

Assessment stresses that every individual action is important. It says, "The choices people make on a day-to-day basis—how to power homes and businesses, get around, and produce and use food and other goods—collectively determine the amount of greenhouse gases emitted."[38]

In the United States transportation-related emissions are the biggest cause of climate change–causing greenhouse gases, so people can help improve the air by changing the way they get around. PeopleForBikes, an organization that encourages people to ride bicycles, reports that most of the daily trips that people take are less than 3 miles (4.8 km) and argues that riding a bike on at least some of those trips instead of taking a car can do a lot to reduce emissions. The group explains, "According to a study conducted in Europe, if 10% of the population were to replace one car trip a day with a bike ride, overall carbon emissions from transportation would drop an equal 10%."[39] In addition, the same study also revealed that a person's transportation-related emis-

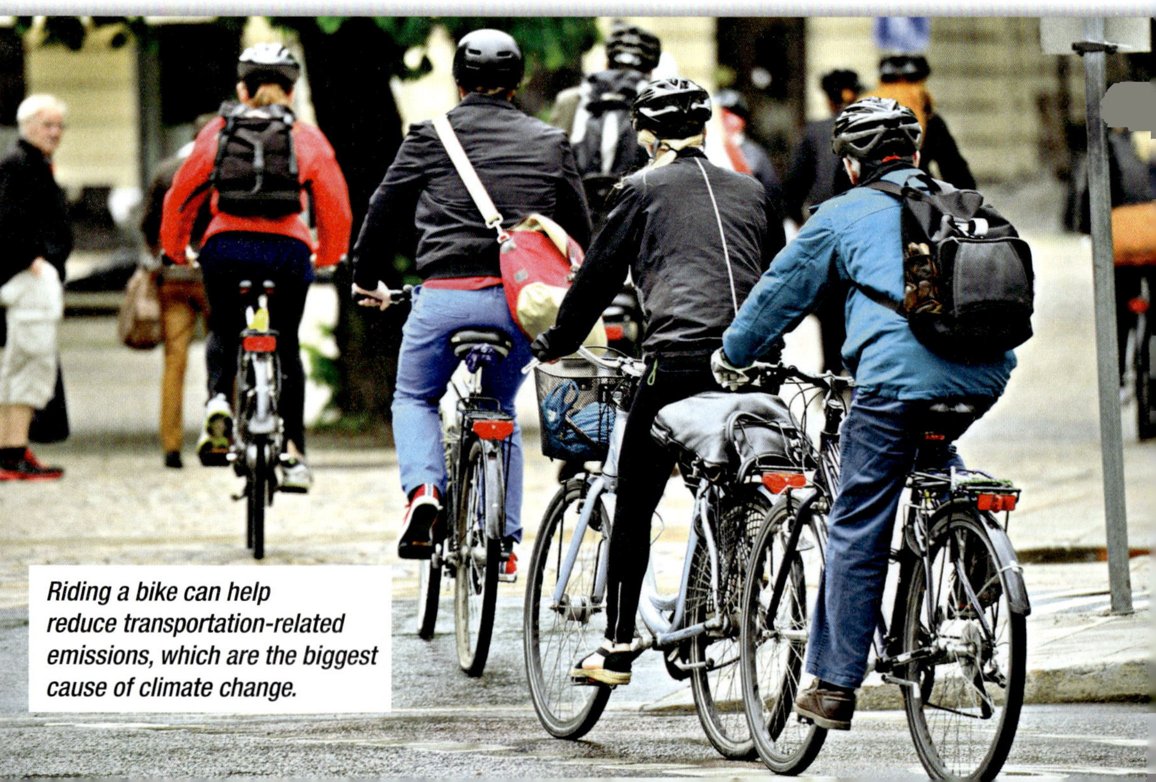

Riding a bike can help reduce transportation-related emissions, which are the biggest cause of climate change.

sions could be reduced by 67 percent if he or she chose to ride a bike just once a day instead of driving.

There is evidence that it is possible to significantly improve air quality in even the most polluted cities. For instance, the Clean Air Fund, a global organization that works to improve air quality around the world, shares the story of Ulaanbaatar, the capital city of Mongolia, which has made significant air quality improvements in the past few years. The Clean Air Fund explains, "In 2022, the average $PM_{2.5}$ [particulate matter of less than 2.5 micrometers in size] levels [were] eleven times higher than the daily WHO recommended limits. But in 2018, the average particulate matter pollution levels were almost 40 times higher than the daily WHO limits."[40] The group says that this dramatic reduction in pollution was achieved through a combination of government commitment to clean air and international funding from organizations like the World Bank. Ulaanbaatar's story is just one of many examples around the world that show people do not have to resign themselves to a future of polluted air.

CHAPTER THREE

The Effects of Extreme Weather Events on Health

In February 2023 Cyclone Freddy ravaged southeast Africa for more than a month. It broke records both for its strength and for how far it traveled. The country of Mozambique was struck once, and then again two weeks later as Freddy circled back. NPR correspondent Kate Bartlett says:

> I spoke to people who had spent days up trees or clinging to roofs to avoid the flood waters, eating leaves to survive. Many children didn't know where their parents were, and there were parents desperately searching for children. One rescued woman said people in her area had been eaten by crocodiles, and a foreign aid worker told me what haunted him most was the survivors' rotting feet—from days of standing in water.[41]

In the end the cyclone killed hundreds of people and sickened or injured many others. It is just one example of how an extreme weather event can impact human health.

Climate Change Means More Extreme Weather

As the world's climate changes, precipitation patterns and temperatures around the world are also changing, and this is causing extreme weather events to occur more often. As an example, the EPA finds that the United States today receives more of its precipitation in intense single-day events than in previous decades. The agency says, "The prevalence of extreme single-day precipitation events remained fairly steady between 1910 and the 1980s but has risen substantially since then. Nationwide, nine of the top 10 years for extreme one-day precipitation events have occurred since 1996."[42]

Similarly, the National Aeronautics and Space Administration (NASA) warns, "As Earth's climate changes, it is impacting extreme weather across the planet. Record-breaking heat waves on land and in the ocean, drenching rains, severe floods, years-long droughts, extreme wildfires, and widespread flooding during hurricanes are all becoming more frequent and more intense."[43] According to a

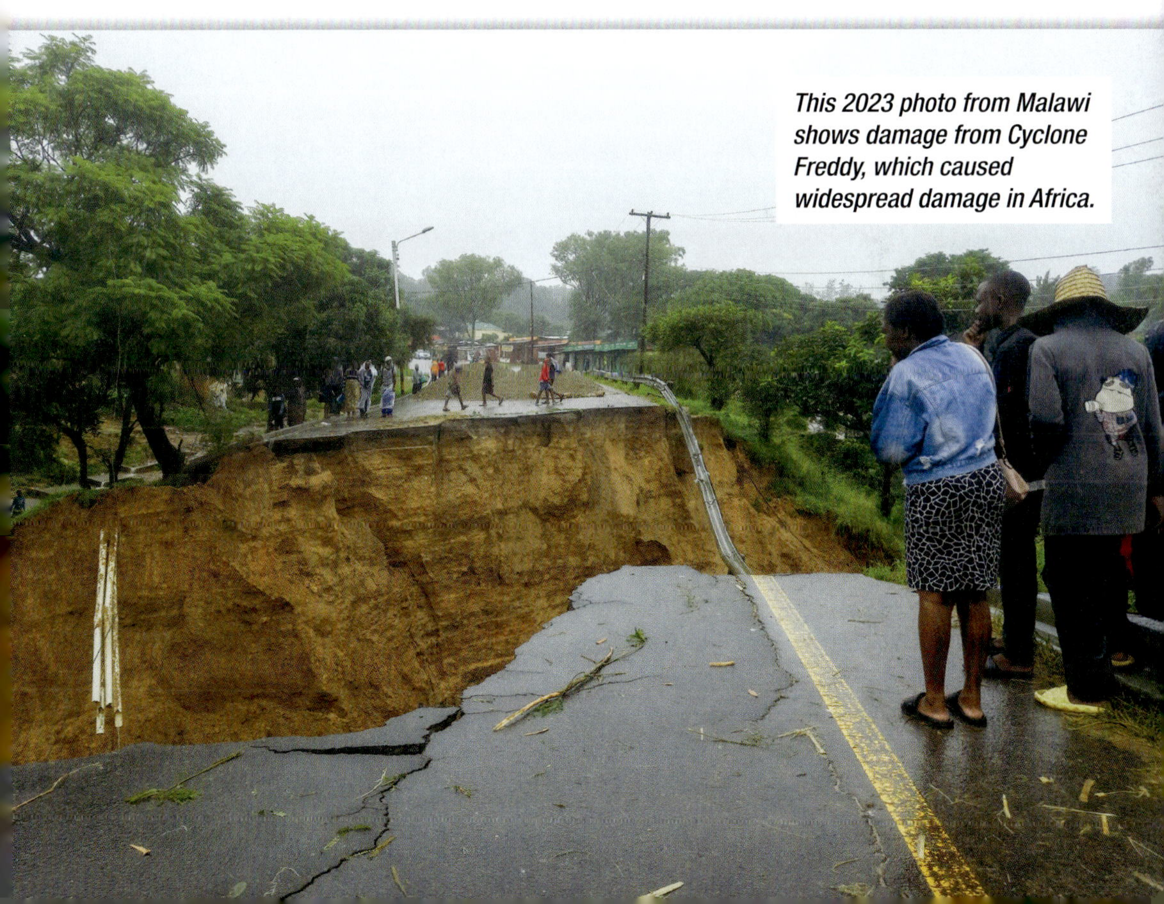

This 2023 photo from Malawi shows damage from Cyclone Freddy, which caused widespread damage in Africa.

2023 Gallup poll, one in three Americans had been personally affected by extreme weather in the previous two years. NASA predicts that as the climate continues to warm, all of these types of extreme weather events will become even more common.

Extreme events are often devastating to human health because people are not prepared for them. Climate scientist Gavin Schmidt explains:

We have systems and infrastructure in place that help us deal with the climate that we had. But climate is changing. We are pushing our living space into areas, into temperatures that we have never experienced. . . . We are moving out of society's comfort zone. And that means that places that were prepared for a certain spread of temperature and a certain number of extremes are now being hit with larger extremes.[44]

The problem with these extremes, he says, is that society's infrastructure has not been designed to handle them. This means that an extreme weather event can also cause extreme devastation.

How Extreme Weather Harms Human Health

Extreme weather events affect human health in a variety of ways. One is that people can be injured or die either during the extreme event itself or in their attempt to escape that event. One example of this is the extreme flooding that occurred in northern India in August 2023. Unusually heavy rain produced floods that washed away roads and buildings and killed more than seventy people. Many of these people died because they were buried in mud or in buildings that collapsed. According to a BBC report, a temple in the town of Shimla collapsed and was buried in a landslide, killing twenty people, including seven members of one family. Sanjay Thakur, who lost his seventeen-year-old son Saurabh in this landslide, says, "We heard the sound of a thunder that morning. . . . I saw that the building had fallen partially. A person stuck in debris was shouting for help. . . . We quickly rushed to rescue him. Then another landslide took place and earth from the rail tracks above the temple came down washing the temple away. There was nothing left."[45]

In 2023 Greece also received record rainfall, with up to 30 inches (76.2 cm) falling in one day in some places. This led to widespread flooding, and according to news reports, at least fifteen people died and dozens were injured. Store owner Erkan Gurer recalls how powerless he felt in the face of so much water. He says, "We came here after our neighbors called us. When we got here, there was water up to the ceiling of our store. There was nothing we could do. We were helpless."[46] Another resident, Vasilis Batsios, says, "This has never happened before here. There was a lot of water, and for many hours. For 24 hours, it was nonstop. The amount of water was unbelievable."[47]

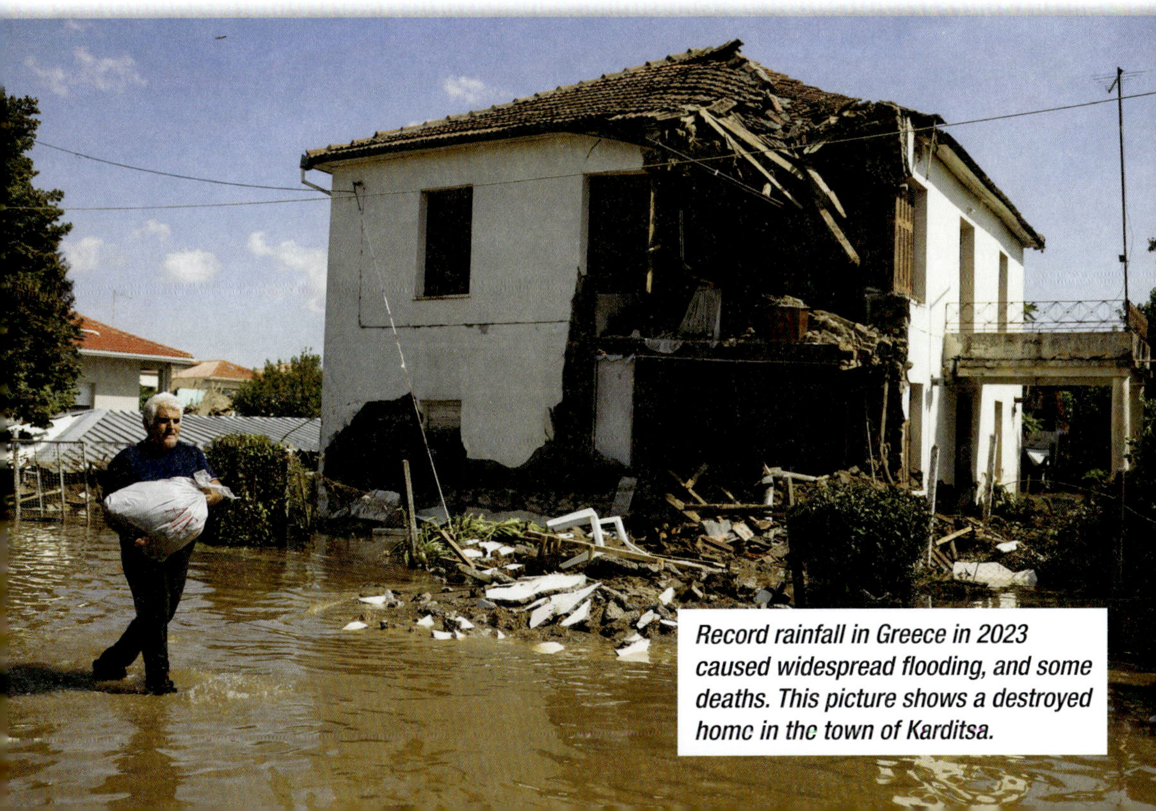

Record rainfall in Greece in 2023 caused widespread flooding, and some deaths. This picture shows a destroyed home in the town of Karditsa.

Extreme events damage homes and other essential infrastructure, and people's health can be negatively affected when they are left without shelter, sanitation, food, clean water, health care, or other things they need to stay healthy. For example, when Cyclone Freddy swept through Africa, hospitals were both damaged by the storm and overwhelmed by the demand for medical attention, leaving many people without access to care. In addition, the cyclone damaged water supply systems, and a lack of clean water led to the spread of cholera in some areas.

Damage caused by extreme weather events can produce long-term negative effects. For example, the CDC explains that flood damage can cause health problems months or years later. It says:

> Water intrusion into buildings can result in mold contamination that manifests later, leading to indoor air quality problems. . . . Populations living in damp indoor environments experience increased prevalence of asthma and other upper respiratory tract symptoms, such as coughing and wheezing, as well as lower respiratory tract infections such as pneumonia, respiratory syncytial virus (RSV), and RSV pneumonia.[48]

Effects of Flooding

Flooding actually has some benefits to the ecosystem. Floodwater can carry organic material and nutrients like nitrogen, leaving them behind on flooded areas, where they act as fertilizer and can help plants grow better. Floods can also increase groundwater supplies. *National Geographic* explains, "Floodwater gets absorbed into the ground then percolates through layers of soil and rock, eventually reaching underground aquifers. These aquifers supply clean freshwater to springs, wells, lakes, and rivers." However, flooding can also be harmful, particularly when it is frequent and severe, as it is predicted to become with climate change. Severe floods can kill people and displace them from their homes. Flooding can cause water supplies to become contaminated by runoff, making them unsafe to drink, and it can also overwhelm sanitation systems, thereby spreading contagious diseases.

National Geographic, "The Many Effects of Flooding." https://education.nationalgeographic.org.

After Hurricane Ida swept through parts of the United States in 2021, Charlene Dionio, who lives in New Jersey, experienced some of the health problems that can come from extreme weather. She says that the water from the storm caused mold to grow in her house, which affected her and her family, particularly her father, who already had health issues from chronic obstructive pulmonary disease. She says that she and her daughter had allergic reactions, but for her father, the health consequences were more severe. "We're healthy and we started having symptoms," she says, "When he's exposed, when he inhales it, with his age and his condition, it will just balloon or mushroom into something that he cannot tolerate."[49] The mold growth after the hurricane left Dionio's father unable to breathe adequately, and he had to spend three days in the hospital.

Extreme Events and Mental Trauma

In addition to physical harm, the many traumatic experiences that often occur during these extreme events—such as displacement from homes, loss of possessions, and even loss of friends and family members—can cause mental health issues. The American Psychiatric Association explains that these traumas can result in depression, anxiety, post-traumatic stress disorder, and even suicide. It says, "Children are more affected by disasters than adults and are more likely to have continued trauma-related symptoms after a disaster. . . . Disruptions in routine, separation from caregivers as a result of evacuations or displacement, and parental stress after a disaster all contribute to children's distress."[50] In addition, the organization says, first responders and emergency workers are also prone to developing mental health problems after extreme events because they often witness multiple deaths and injuries, and they may have to juggle caring for the public with looking after their own friends or family members.

There are many examples of mental trauma resulting from extreme events. In 2021 Texas endured a period of extreme winter cold, and some people lost power for days. San Antonio resident

Health Care Costs of Extreme Events

According to a recent report made by the US Senate Committee on the Budget, the health care costs of extreme weather and other types of climate change are substantial and rising. As an example, the report points to Hurricane Sandy, which occurred in 2012: "Hurricane Sandy is estimated to have cost $3.3 billion in health costs—this included nearly 4700 emergency room visits, over 6600 hospital admissions, and 273 deaths." The US Department of the Treasury notes that certain groups of people are more likely to experience financial strain as a result of weather-related expenses, including lower-income people who often lack health insurance, as well as people already suffering from health conditions. In addition, the department says:

> Climate hazards can exacerbate existing health inequities for households that are underserved by healthcare resources. In particular, households in rural or lower-income areas already have limited healthcare services. When climate hazards further reduce access in these areas, households may experience delayed treatment or management of healthcare conditions, which could lead to adverse health outcomes and increased healthcare costs over the longer-term.

US Senate Committee on the Budget, "Whitehouse: Climate Change Is Driving Up Health Care Costs, Dragging Down Economic Growth," April 24, 2023. www.budget.senate.gov.

US Department of the Treasury, "The Impact of Climate Change on American Household Finances," 2023. https://home.treasury.gov.

Kim Mair describes how the experience traumatized her. She said the freeze was a disaster for her family and explains that she now has anxiety about the power going out whenever the temperature begins to drop. The threat of extreme cold returned in 2023, and she says, "When I heard some people say it was snowing by them, it was dread. Instead of it being happiness and excitement, it was dread. . . . How many people are going to die this time?"[51]

Luca Maxwell Gibreath, an Austin resident, fell and hurt himself during the 2021 storm, leaving him with a disability that makes it difficult to walk. "I won't say I'm traumatized by the ice now, but it does make me hypervigilant and over-cautious about going outside," he says. "I don't want to go out, but my dogs need walks, so they've been keeping me going out and facing it."[52]

Fighting Back Against Nature

As extreme weather events become more prevalent, a growing number of people are recognizing that rather than trying to live the same way they always have, communities need to accept that these events will occur and take steps to be prepared when they do. An example of this type of adaptation occurred in Iowa City, Iowa, after flooding in 2008 inundated a large wastewater treatment plant near the river. Rather than simply rebuilding the plant, the city recognized that climate change would make another flood likely and decided to decommission the plant and move operations to an area outside of the floodplain. The EPA explains, "By decommissioning the vulnerable wastewater treatment plant and converting the surrounding area into a public greenspace, the city adapts to reduce the threat and impact of future extreme storm events."[53]

In Seattle, Washington, an entire village is relocating as a way to reduce the future harms of extreme weather. The Quinault Indian Nation village of Taholah is located about 150 miles (241 km) west of Seattle. It has experienced massive flooding resulting

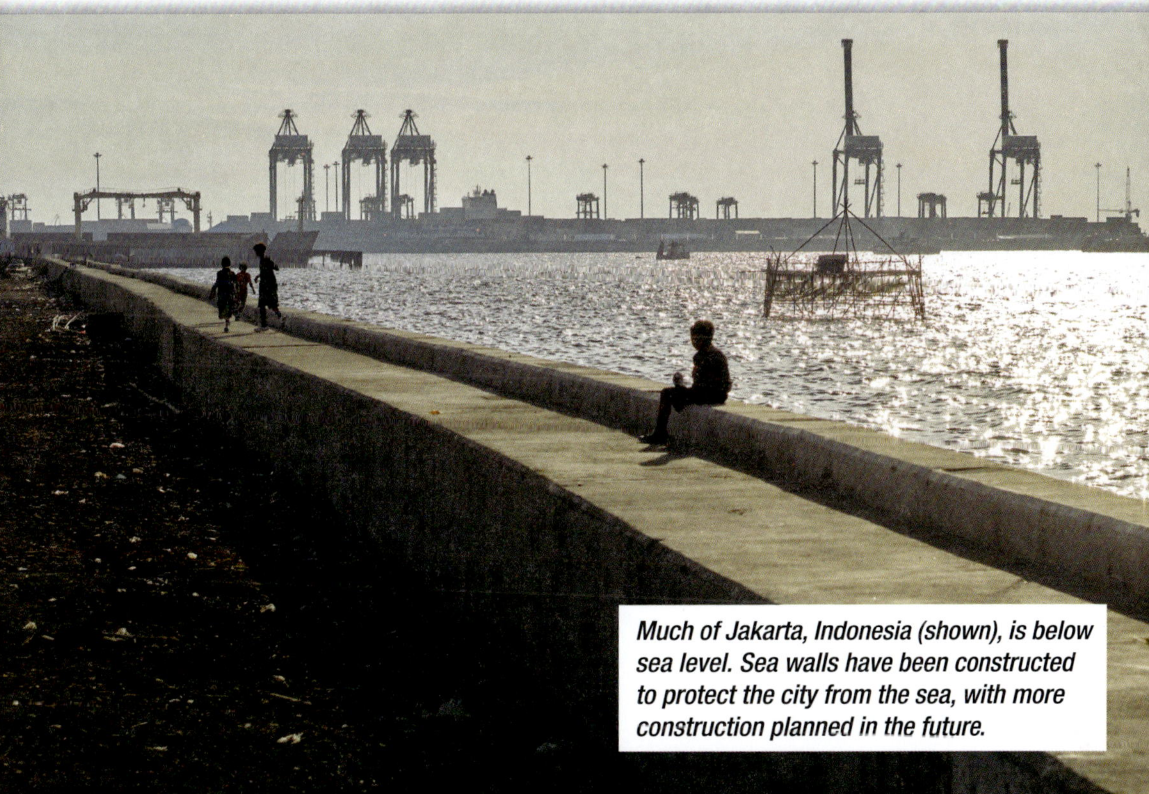

Much of Jakarta, Indonesia (shown), is below sea level. Sea walls have been constructed to protect the city from the sea, with more construction planned in the future.

from sea level rise and extreme weather events. Lia Frenchman, who lives in Taholah, says, "I've never seen this type of flooding in my lifetime. . . . When it does flood, unfortunately, my end of the street has a large dip in the road and the water will stay for up to a week at a time. And so I'm basically either trapped or not able to come home."[54] After studying the situation, the Quinault Indian Nation has made plans to relocate Taholah to nearby tribal land at a higher elevation. It received a $25 million grant from the US Department of the Interior to help it do so.

Other low-lying communities whose size make it impractical to relocate have built large sea walls to protect themselves. One example is the city of Jakarta in Indonesia. According to *National Geographic*, approximately 40 percent of the city is currently below sea level, and the situation is rapidly becoming worse. The publication explains that the area has plans to substantially alter the landscape to protect its people from the rising seas. It says, "A 'Giant Sea Wall' is to be constructed offshore in Jakarta Bay. It's to include a 20-mile-long artificial island in the shape of a bird—the Garuda, Indonesia's national symbol. The 10,000-acre island will block storm surges, but it is also supposed to house offices and apartments, a water reservoir, highways and train tracks, as well as recreational facilities."[55] All around the world, people are coming to similar realizations that they are not powerless in the face of nature's extreme weather, and they are creating innovative solutions such as this to adapt to a future in which extreme events will be more common.

CHAPTER FOUR

Vector-Borne Diseases and Human Health

Malaria is a serious and potentially fatal disease that is spread through mosquito bites. It is very prevalent in some parts of the world, including Africa and areas in Asia and South America, where it has caused millions of illnesses and hundreds of thousands of deaths. In the United States it is rare, and most cases occur among people who caught the disease while traveling to places where it is common. That may be changing. In 2023 Florida resident Hannah Heath—who had not left the country—developed a fever and chills and was throwing up. She says that at first she thought she had food poisoning, but she rapidly became sicker. She says, "Finally I called my husband and I was like, 'You have to take me to the ER, I think I'm dehydrated; I think I need an IV.'" At the hospital, doctors told her that she had malaria. "I was like, 'You're kidding me, right?'" she says, "Because I haven't been outside the country, so it was just surreal."[56]

Heath was one of eight people in Texas and Florida who caught malaria within the United States in 2023, the first time this has happened in twenty years. As the climate warms, the range and life spans of mosquitoes and other organisms that spread diseases to people are changing, and so are the health risks posed by these organisms. This means that some parts of the world are likely to see a variety of new health threats.

How Climate Change Affects Disease-Causing Vectors

Malaria is caused by a parasite that infects people through the bites of infected mosquitoes. It is known as a vector-borne disease, which is a disease that is spread from one host to another by an organism like a mosquito, tick, or flea, which are officially referred to as vectors. Vector-borne diseases occur all over the world; however, the diseases vary by area since every vector needs a specific climate in which to live and breed. Mosquitoes cause the largest number of vector-borne diseases, including malaria, West Nile virus, Zika, dengue, and chikungunya. Ticks also cause vector-borne diseases, including Lyme disease and tick-borne encephalitis. Other vector-borne diseases include sleeping sickness, caused by tsetse flies; leishmaniasis, caused by sand flies; typhus, caused by lice; and Chagas disease, caused by triatomine bugs. Many vector-borne diseases lead to serious health problems and are often fatal.

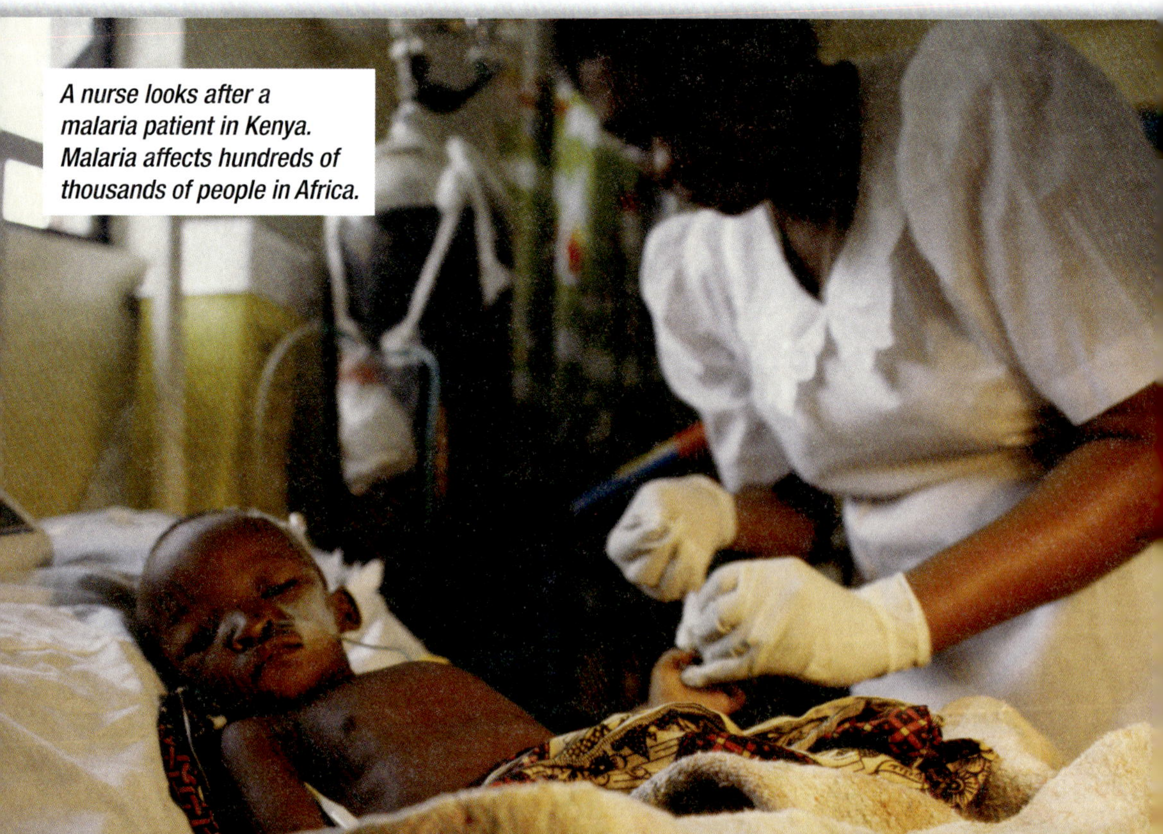

A nurse looks after a malaria patient in Kenya. Malaria affects hundreds of thousands of people in Africa.

Vectors generally live in warm climates, and as the world gets warmer, researchers are finding that vectors are able to live in more parts of the world than they have previously. Warmer weather also means that many vectors can live and breed for longer periods. The CDC explains, "Because warmer average temperatures can mean longer warm seasons, earlier spring seasons, shorter and milder winters, and hotter summers, conditions might become more hospitable for many carriers of vector-borne diseases."[57] As an example, the CDC reports that in the United States, the geographic range of ticks, fleas, and mosquitoes has expanded over time. Similar expansions have also been observed in other countries. In addition, climate change threatens to cause the emergence of new vector-borne illnesses. In the United States alone, the CDC reports that nine new vector-borne viruses and parasites have been identified since 2004.

The impact of climate change on vectors is not all positive. While rising temperatures mean that vectors can expand to new areas, some areas are also growing too warm for the vectors that live there. However, as with most other effects of climate change, researchers are finding that the negative impacts far outweigh the positive; the overall trend worldwide is an increase in vector habitats.

Vector-Borne Diseases and Human Health

As the vector population expands its reach and grows in size, people are at increased risk of being harmed by vector-borne diseases. In a 2022 study in *Nature Climate Change*, researchers explain that a significant number of infectious diseases are being affected by climate change. They state, "We found that 58% (that is, 218 out of 375) of infectious diseases confronted by humanity worldwide have been at some point aggravated by climatic hazards."[58] The CDC also reports that vector-borne diseases are a growing problem. In a 2020 report, it says, "During the last 15 years, the number of vector-borne disease cases has increased dramatically as the ranges of vectors have expanded and the number of emerging pathogens have multiplied." It finds that in the United States and its territories, between 2004 and 2018, the number of vector-borne diseases in people doubled. Overall, the CDC concludes, "What is certain is that more pathogens put more Americans at risk. More people at risk."[59]

One example of the spread of disease-causing vectors as a result of climate change is the expansion of ticks in North America. Ticks are sensitive to temperature, and warmer temperatures mean that they can survive in a wider range of places. The EPA says, "Studies provide evidence that climate change has contributed to the expanded range of ticks . . . such as in areas of Canada where the ticks were previously unable to survive."[60] In the United States the EPA reports that the most common vector-borne disease is Lyme disease, spread by the bite of a tick, which affects at least twenty thousand to thirty thousand people per year. Research

West Nile Virus in the United States

In the United States, West Nile virus is the most common mosquito-borne disease, and case numbers are growing as a result of climate change. While many people have no symptoms after being infected with West Nile virus, it causes serious illness in others. The EPA explains, "[People] can experience symptoms such as headache, body aches, joint pains, vomiting, diarrhea, and rash, as well as more severe damage to the central nervous system in some patients, causing encephalitis, meningitis, and occasionally death." The agency reports that there were more than fifty-five thousand cases of West Nile virus in the United States during 1999 to 2021. It also has found that climate change can cause mosquitoes to grow faster, bite more, and be more likely to incubate West Nile virus, all of which means that climate change is increasing the risk of human exposure to the disease in the United States.

US Environmental Protection Agency, "Climate Change Indicators: West Nile Virus," October 13, 2023. www.epa.gov.

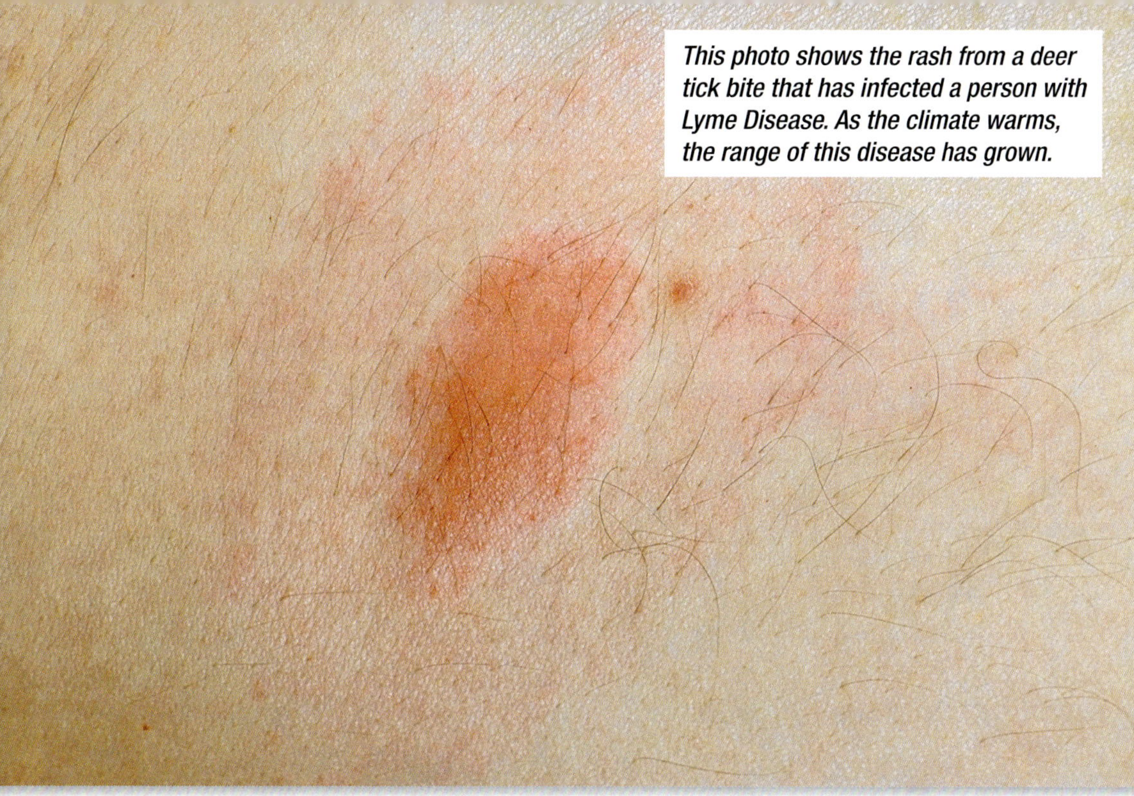

shows that over the past twenty years, cases of Lyme disease and other tick-borne illnesses, including Rocky Mountain spotted fever, have increased in the United States. According to the EPA, "The incidence of Lyme disease in the United States has nearly doubled since 1991, from 3.74 reported cases per 100,000 people to 7.21 reported cases per 100,000 people in 2018."[61] The EPA reports that the biggest increases have been in Maine and Vermont.

Lyme disease is also occurring in places where it was not found in the past. Vishnu Laalitha Surapaneni, an assistant professor of internal medicine at the University of Minnesota Medical School, says, "We're observing that the tick is moving more into Canada." In addition, she says, "We also see Lyme disease cases in Norway, as well as in the Arctic."[62] Lyme disease can cause fever, fatigue, joint pain, and nervous system problems.

CONSIDER THIS

Since 1991 cases of Lyme disease have almost doubled in the United States.

—US Environmental Protection Agency

Benjamin Beard, deputy director of the CDC's division of vector-borne diseases, says, "Lyme disease is . . . a very serious disease. . . . People have even died from early Lyme disease. . . . If you don't pick it up early and it becomes disseminated in your body, . . . it can become much more difficult to treat."[63]

Mosquito-Borne Illnesses

In addition to tick-borne illnesses, mosquito-borne illnesses are becoming an increasing threat as the climate changes. The World Mosquito Program, a nonprofit group that is working to protect people from mosquito-borne diseases, stresses that illnesses caused by mosquitoes are already a significant problem in many parts of the world. It says that these diseases kill more than a million people and infect up to 700 million people a year, which equates to one person for every ten in the world. It warns that what is already a significant health threat will only become worse as the climate changes, saying, "As the planet warms and climate change lengthens the mosquito season, the world's deadliest creature will expand its geographical range to new regions and re-emerge in areas where mosquito numbers had subsided for decades."[64]

In a study published in the *Lancet* in 2021, researchers agree that climate change is increasing the threat of mosquito-borne illnesses. They report that climate change will enable mosquitoes to survive longer and to broaden their range. The researchers conclude that the health consequences of these changes will be significant: "The population at risk of [malaria and dengue fever] might increase by up to 4.7 additional billion people by 2070 relative to 1970–99, particularly in lowlands and urban areas."[65] Similarly, the World Mosquito Program states, "the Early Warning System for Mosquito Borne Diseases (EYWA) shows an upward trajectory in Europe, with malaria cases increasing by 62% and dengue, Zika and chikungunya by 700%." It goes on to explain that Southern Australia is also seeing a rising mosquito problem: "The region is

In some places climate change is reducing vector activity instead of increasing it. One such place is the Zambezi valley in Zimbabwe. Temperatures in this area have risen so much in recent years that tsetse fly populations are smaller than ever before. Tsetse flies are the vector for sleeping sickness, a potentially fatal disease, and one study shows that rates of sleeping sickness have declined in the Zambezi valley. However, tsetse flies are not disappearing altogether. Instead, researchers have found that they are migrating north, to areas that were previously too cold for them to live.

currently grappling with its first major outbreak of Japanese encephalitis, a mosquito-transmitted infection more commonly found in rural southeast Asia and the Pacific Islands. Scientists believe climate change has potentially created a 'perfect storm,' allowing the virus to move further south and gain a foothold in the country."[66]

While mosquitoes transmit many diseases, malaria is the most common worldwide. It causes flu-like symptoms, including sweats, chills, body aches, and nausea. Untreated, malaria can cause seizures and other serious neurological symptoms and can be life threatening. According to microbiologist Laura Norris, who has spent seventeen years studying this disease, "In 2021, there were an estimated 247 million malaria cases, including 619,000 deaths."[67] She says that 95 percent of these cases were in Africa, and three-quarters of deaths were in children under age five.

Dengue fever is another disease transmitted by mosquitoes. In some cases this illness is relatively mild, but it can be extremely painful and dangerous. Georgie Darling, who lived in Indonesia and suffered from dengue fever, recalls her experience:

I watched, in agony, as my body struggled to cope. A splitting headache exploded across my temples and refused to waver. The aches were akin to the most intense workout—and then some. Sickness and nausea left me incapable of doing any more than sipping rehydration drinks or sucking ginger sweets. I was five days into this when I tried to sit up in bed and experienced stomach pains so severe that they made me cry out, tears streaming down my face. I called the hospital. . . . I spent days in and out of fevers, shivering and vomiting.[68]

Addressing the Threat of Vector-Borne Diseases

Although climate change is accelerating the threat of vector-borne diseases in many parts of the world, there are also several innovative efforts to reduce this threat. Some companies have focused on developing new treatments for vector-borne diseases. The Drugs for Neglected Diseases initiative (DNDi) stresses that these diseases disproportionally affect poor and vulnerable communities, and the initiative works to develop new treatments specifically for these communities. It gives one example of a recent success story in South Asia, where it has helped develop an improved treatment for a tropical disease called visceral leishmaniasis, or kala-azar, which is transmitted through sand fly bites. DNDi says, "Until recently, the only treatment for kala-azar was a . . . painful series of injections, which required a hospital stay and close monitoring of patients for potentially fatal side effects. Clinical trials carried out by DNDi and partners in India proved the effectiveness of a single-dose infusion. It is also safer for patients and easier for healthcare workers."[69] According to DNDi, without treatment, kala-azar is almost always fatal, but due to this new treatment, the number of people suffering because of this disease in South Asia has declined from thirty thousand in 2005 to only about two thousand in 2020.

Some researchers think that they can use genetic engineering to modify vectors and thereby reduce the threat of vector-borne diseases. For example, this technology could be used to modify mosquitoes so that they cannot transmit malaria. *New York Times* journalist Stephanie Nolen explains that several different groups are

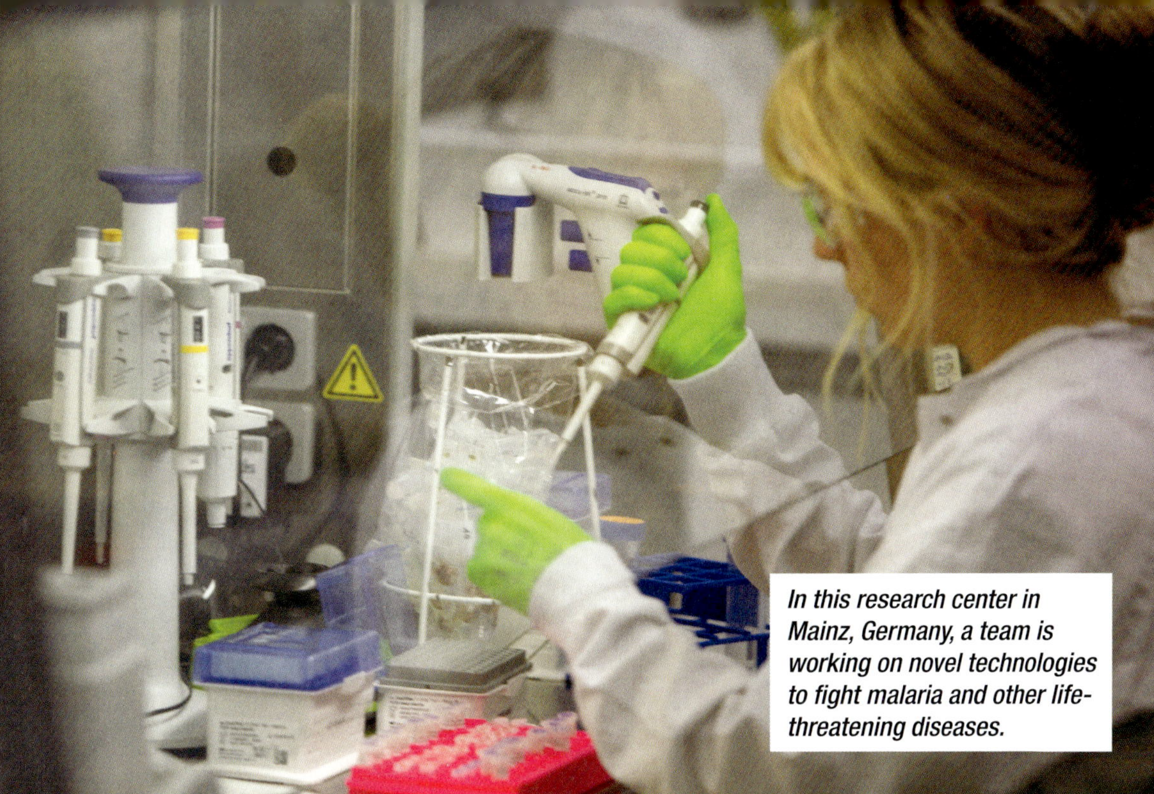

In this research center in Mainz, Germany, a team is working on novel technologies to fight malaria and other life-threatening diseases.

currently working on doing this, all using slightly different strategies. She describes one group of researchers working on genetic engineering of mosquitoes on an island off the coast of Africa, saying, "Their idea is to release a small colony of genetically modified mosquitoes . . . to mate with wild ones. The gene engineering technology they are using could, in just a few generations—a matter of months when it comes to mosquitoes—make every member of the species that transmits malaria here, the Anopheles coluzzii, effectively immune to the parasite [that causes malaria]."[70] Greg Lanzaro, a molecular geneticist who is the leader of the team, believes that the group is close to success. He says, "We've been working on this for 30 years. . . . And we believe we have it."[71]

This technology is not without controversy though. Critics worry that it could have unintended effects, like causing unforeseen harm to the ecosystem. Genetic engineering is just one way that people are working to reduce the threat that vector-borne diseases pose to society, and many researchers are optimistic that ultimately, many innovative solutions to the threat of such diseases will be invented.

CHAPTER FIVE

The Health Consequences of Changing Water Quality

Few living things can exist without water. Water moves around the earth and the atmosphere in a complex process called the water cycle. It falls to the ground as rain or snow, where it is absorbed into the ground or runs off into bodies of water. At the same time, water also evaporates back into the atmosphere. The process is constant. The water cycle controls where, when, and how water moves, and it happens in a slightly different way in every part of the world. Some locations have an abundance of water, while others have hardly any. Some receive most of their water in the form of rain, while for others it is snow. While these patterns can fluctuate from year to year, for much of human history they have also remained relatively predictable, and around the world people have become accustomed to their water supplies being a certain way. Climate change is altering that. The United Nations explains, "Water and climate change are inextricably linked." As a result of climate change, it says, "[Water is becoming] more scarce, more unpredictable, more polluted or all three."[72] People need clean water for drinking, sanitation, growing crops, and raising animals, and as climate change alters the availability and the quality of the earth's water supplies, people's health is being dramatically affected.

How Climate Change Affects Water Supplies

Most scientists agree that climate change is altering water cycle patterns around the world. The Intergovernmental Panel on Climate Change reports, "All components of the global water cycle have been modified due to climate change in recent decades . . . with hundreds of millions of people now regularly experiencing hydrological conditions that were previously unfamiliar. . . . Records from weather stations, satellites and radar clearly show that precipitation patterns have shifted worldwide."[73] Changes in the global water cycle mean that many people have trouble getting the water they need for drinking, sanitation, and farming.

Water shortages have become ever more common and more pronounced in many parts of the world, including Africa, Australia, China, and the Mediterranean. For example, aid organization Oxfam International explains that in the Horn of Africa, water shortages have become so severe that families are losing the animals in their herds and are forced to constantly keep moving in search of water. Abdilal Yassen, who lives in this area, explains that he has always had to deal with periods when water was scarce, but he says that things have become much worse in the past few years. He explains that the lack of water is forcing animals and people either to move away from the area or to die: "We used to lose some animals, but we would always have food and water. But this is different. It is 'sweeping away' animals and people."[74]

Water has become increasingly scarce in some parts of the United States as well. *The Fifth National Climate Assessment* reports that water shortages have "strained surface water and groundwater supplies, reduced agricultural productivity, and lowered water levels in major reservoirs."[75] Further, it predicts that these water shortages will become more intense, more frequent,

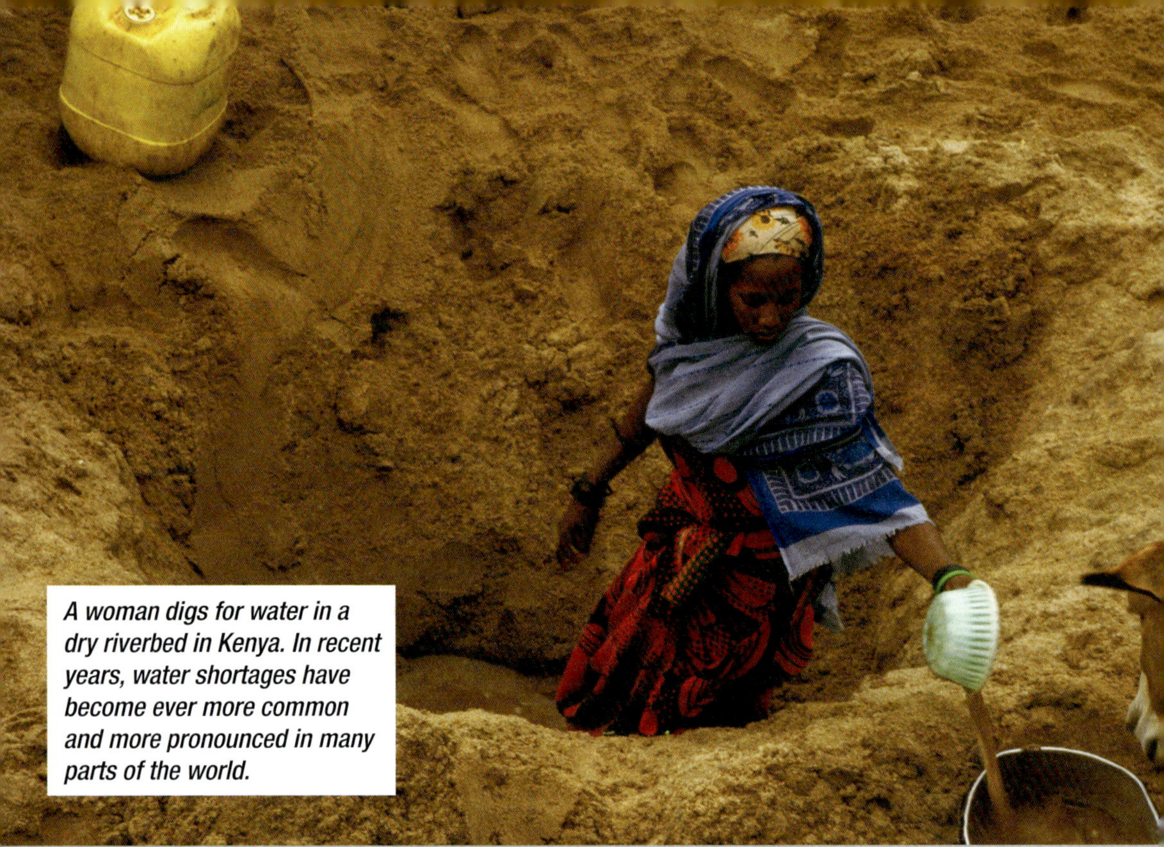

A woman digs for water in a dry riverbed in Kenya. In recent years, water shortages have become ever more common and more pronounced in many parts of the world.

and more long-lasting in the future, in the southwestern United States and in other parts of the country.

Another effect of climate change is that as the climate warms, ice sheets and glaciers are melting, and ocean levels are slowly rising, which is having a negative effect on some water supplies. According to the National Oceanic and Atmospheric Administration (NOAA), the ocean is likely to rise by at least 1 foot (30.5 cm) above 2000 levels by the end of the century. This is threatening water quality in areas near the ocean, through a process called saltwater—or seawater—intrusion. Hydrogeologist Holly Michael explains this process, saying:

I think of seawater intrusion as being like a seesaw: The place where fresh water and salt water meet is the balance point between forces from land and forces from the sea. A push from the land side, such as heavy rainfall or high river flows, moves the balance point seaward. A push from the sea side—whether it's sea-level rise, storm surge or high tides—moves the balance point landward. Droughts or heavy use of fresh water can also cause seawater to move inland.[76]

This seesaw happens in both groundwater supplies and in rivers that flow into the ocean. In recent years there has been increasing saltwater intrusion in many parts of the world.

Warming Water and Contaminants

Another way climate change is affecting water supplies is that many bodies of water are becoming warmer, leading to an increase in certain harmful contaminants that flourish there. Harmful algal blooms are one example. Algae are a type of plant that lives in both fresh water and salt water. While some algae are beneficial to marine environments, other types release toxins. People and animals who drink or swim in water contaminated with these

Declining Snowpacks

In many parts of the world, people depend on winter snowpacks for their water supplies. Snow falls in the winter, creating a snowpack in the mountains. When spring comes, that snowpack gradually melts, adding fresh water to rivers and lakes and helping refill water supplies. Sarah Fecht from the Columbia Climate School explains how climate change is altering this.

As the air warms, many areas are receiving more of their precipitation as rain rather than snow. This means less water is being stored for later as snowpack. In addition, the rain actually accelerates the melting of snow that's already on the ground. The lack of snowpack can lead to drier conditions later in the year, which can be bad news for regions that rely on snowmelt to refill their drinking water supplies.

Fecht says that this is already happening in California, which has seen water shortages due to declining snowpacks.

Sarah Fecht, "How Climate Change Impacts Our Water," Columbia Climate School, September 23, 2019. https://news.climate.columbia.edu.

toxins suffer from health problems, including gastrointestinal issues, skin rashes, and even liver damage. The EPA says, "With a changing climate, harmful algal blooms can occur more often, in more fresh or marine waterbodies, and can be more intense."[77]

There is also evidence that climate change is increasing the frequency of health problems caused by vibrio bacteria. These bacteria thrive in warm, brackish marine water and can cause foodborne illness if people consume seafood from that water, or they can get wound infections if they swim in it. The US Department of Agriculture says, "Vibrio exposure may cause mild vomiting, diarrhea, swimmer's ear, or skin infections. However, it can also result in rare but more serious outcomes like sepsis, amputations, and death." The agency predicts that cases of these illnesses will multiply as climate change causes the ocean to continue to warm. It says, "There is evidence this already may be happening. In 2004, a Vibrio outbreak occurred in Alaska, more than 600 miles north of any previously recorded. Once rare in Oregon and Washington, infections now regularly occur there."[78]

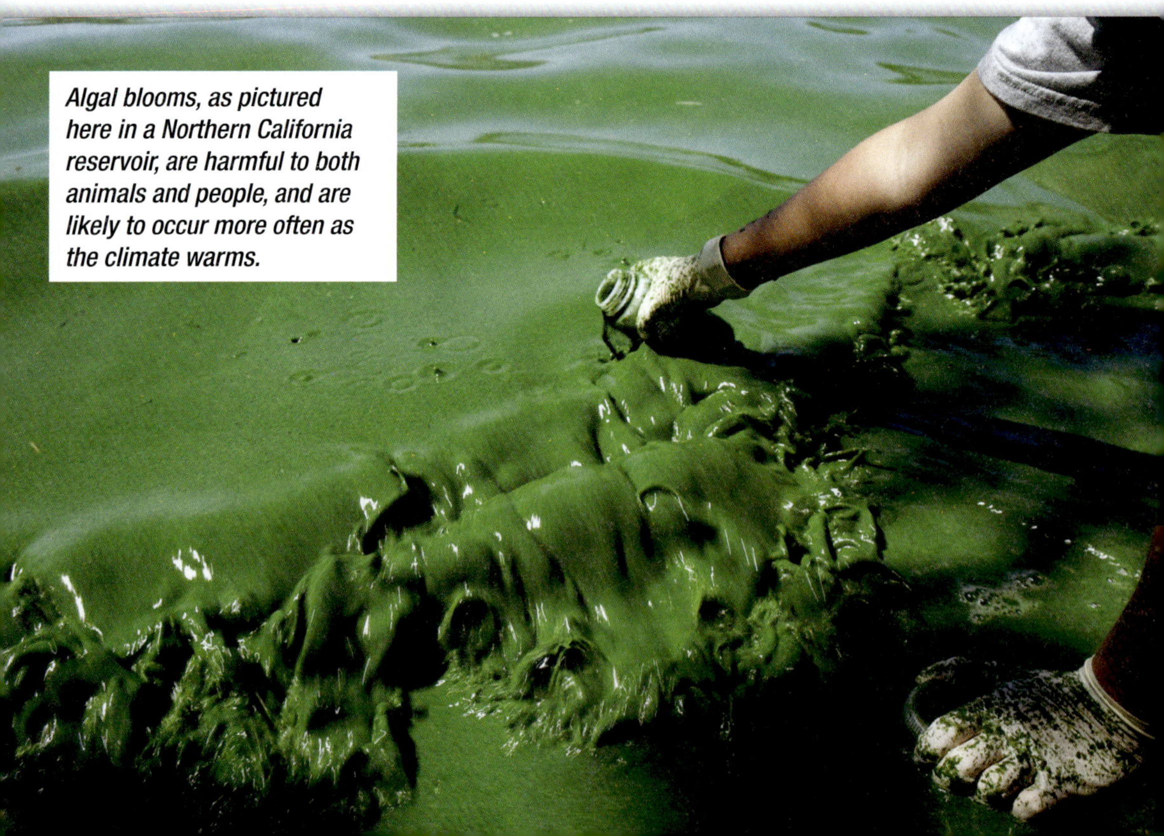

Algal blooms, as pictured here in a Northern California reservoir, are harmful to both animals and people, and are likely to occur more often as the climate warms.

Struggling to Deal with Changes in Water Supplies

All around the world, people's health is being threatened because of the way climate change is altering water supplies. According to news reports, in October 2023 the Amazon's second-largest tributary—the Negro River—was at its lowest level since measurements began 121 years ago, impacting food, water, and sanitation for the people who depend on it. The NOAA says, "Low water levels in the Amazons' tributaries have halted hydroelectric production at Brazil's fourth-largest dam, dried up drinking water, isolated hundreds of communities who depend on rivers for transportation, and led to mass mortality among river dolphins and fish."[79] Caroline Silva dos Santos lives in the Brazilian town of Manacapuru and is one of those people affected by the lack of water. She says, "It is difficult because of the contamination of the water, we need a lot of it to bathe. And we also drink the water, but because it is contaminated we're not drinking it."[80] Fisheman Anesio Junior adds, "The drier it gets, the more fish die and the more precarious the situation becomes."[81]

Another country that is experiencing water-related health threats due to climate change is Kiribati. Some parts of this low-lying island chain are only a few feet above sea level, and many experts predict that the islands will disappear completely within decades. Some areas have already disappeared. For instance, journalist Denise Chow describes the plight of Tebunginako, which she says was once a thriving village: "Beginning in the 1970s, the tide started inching closer to the houses in the village. Over the years, as strong winds whipped up monster waves and climate change caused sea levels to rise, water inundated the

Water Shortages in Malawi

In Malawi more than 1 million people depend on water from Lake Chilwa, the second-largest lake in that country. Sometimes the lake dries up completely, and this greatly disrupts life for all these people. In the past this was very rare; however, today it has become relatively common. Environmental scientist Sosten Chiotha says, "It used to take 25–40 years for natural drying cycles to occur. But now, every three to five years there is an extreme recession in Lake Chilwa. This is the impact of climate change." When the lake dries up, residents of this area are left without drinking water or water for crops and are unable to catch fish, which many rely on for food and to sell to support their families. Alfred Samuel, who lives near the lake, says that in the past he was able to make a good income from selling fish caught in the lake and rice cultivated with lake water. He says, "I now only catch enough fish for my family and my fears are that if the changing climate patterns are not reversed, the lake might completely dry up in the near future."

Quoted in Dennis Lupenga, "Climate Stories: Meet the People Affected by Extreme Weather," WaterAid. www.wateraid.org.

Quoted in Madalitso Wills Kateta, "'Everything Is Changing': The Struggle for Food as Malawi's Lake Chilwa Shrinks," *The Guardian* (Manchester, UK), August 30, 2021. www.the guardian.com.

island, overwhelming a seawall that had been built to protect the community. Barely anything remains of the village today." Speaking to Chow, Kiribati's former president, Anote Tong, adds his own stark description of the village, "It's no longer there. . . . What we do have is a church sitting in the middle of the sea when the tide comes in."[82]

Because the islands are so close to sea level, drinking water in the wells there is becoming contaminated by salt water as the sea rises. Pediatrician Jo Clarke explains that a lack of water to drink is not the only problem this is causing. She says, "A lack of fresh water makes sanitation in the community more difficult, heightens the risk of diarrhea and skin infections, and makes it harder to grow food."[83] In 2022 Kiribati's government declared a state of emergency because this saltwater contamination, in combination with widespread drought, was leaving many residents without enough fresh water.

Most experts predict that the harms of climate change on the water supply will only grow. *The Carbon Almanac* is a collaboration of hundreds of people from more than forty different countries. It reports that one-third of the world's people already do not have access to safe drinking water and insists that climate change will make this situation worse. It says, "By 2050, more than half of the world's population (about five billion), is projected to experience water stress."[84] Water stress is defined as a situation in which there is not enough water to meet demand.

Managing Water Supplies

Climate change threatens water quality around the world; however, water can also be a weapon against the effects of climate change. The United Nations states, "Water can fight climate change." It explains that by taking action to manage water supplies in a sustainable way, communities can help protect themselves from the effects of climate change: "Sustainable water management helps society adapt to climate change by building resilience, protecting health and saving lives. It also mitigates climate change itself by protecting ecosystems and reducing carbon emissions from water and sanitation transportation and treatment."[85]

One suggested sustainable water management strategy is the harvesting of rainwater to store when it is plentiful for use during dry periods. Yemen is one country that is doing this. The World Bank explains that Yemen is one of the most water-scarce countries in the world and that for many people there, finding safe drinking water is a daily challenge. The organization recently worked with three different Yemeni communities to help change that. The communities built cisterns that collect water from roofs and other non-porous surfaces. According to the World Bank, the results have been life-changing for many people who previously had to travel long distances to obtain water. Ali Bakrit, who lives in one of these communities, says, "Sometimes we were left without water for days, but now that problem is gone; this is a dream come true."[86]

For coastal areas that are threatened by sea level rise, some researchers are advocating the creation of what is called a living shoreline. The NOAA explains, "A living shoreline is a protected, stabilized coastal edge made of natural materials such as plants, sand, or rock. Unlike a concrete seawall or other hard structure, which impede[s] the growth of plants and animals, living shorelines grow over time."[87] Living shorelines have many benefits. There is evidence that they are resistant to flooding and erosion. They also help purify water, store carbon, and provide a habitat for wildlife. Denise Maples lives along the Elizabeth River in Chesapeake Bay, Maryland. She created a living shoreline on her property in 2019 and has seen multiple benefits since then, in contrast to neighbors without such a shoreline. The Chesapeake Bay Foundation shares her success story, explaining, "While Denise's property had long been shrinking, it is now gaining back land as the na-

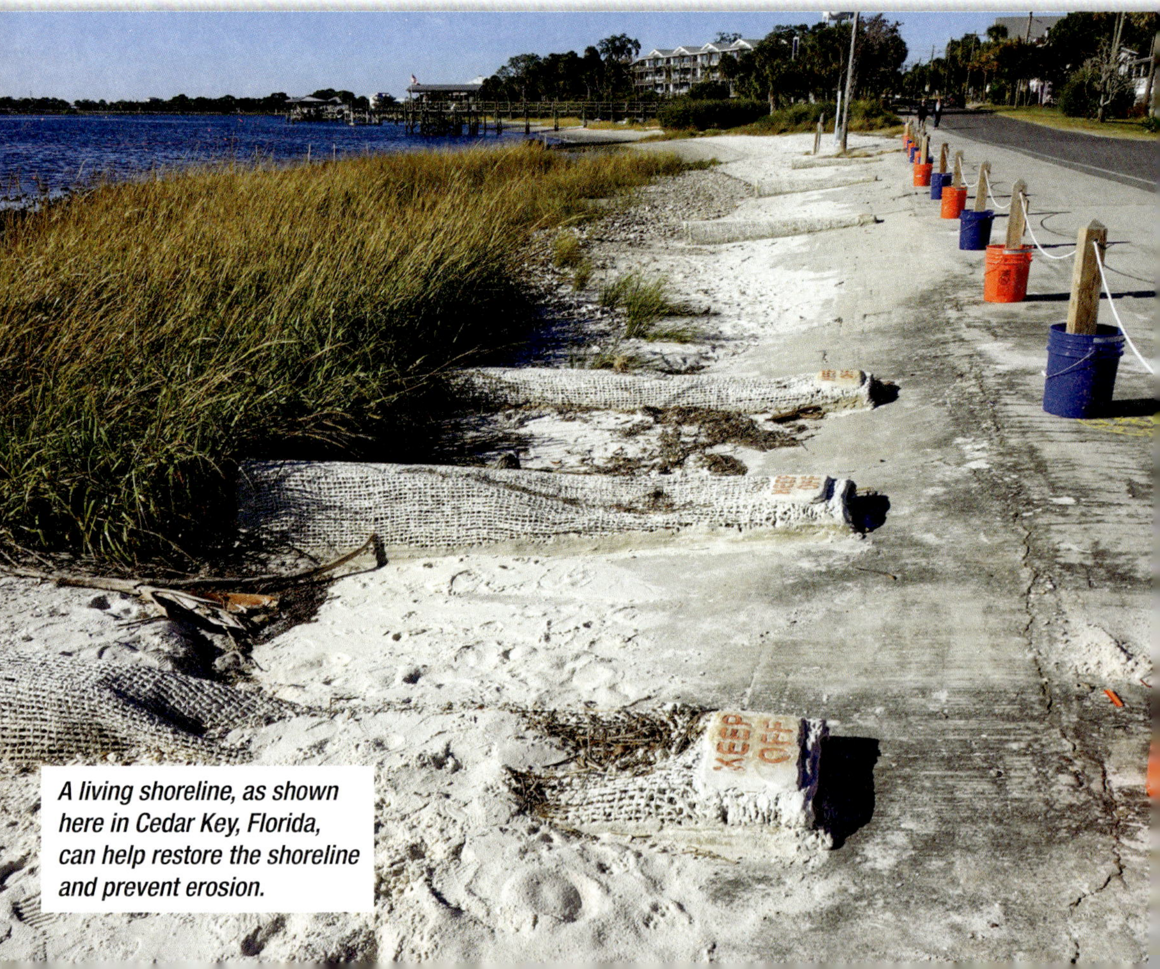

A living shoreline, as shown here in Cedar Key, Florida, can help restore the shoreline and prevent erosion.

tive plants trap sand washed in by the current. Wildlife abounds, from night herons and egrets to foxes and raccoons that forage in the oyster reef at low tide."[88]

Managing water supplies is just one way that society can take action to protect its health in the face of a changing climate. A variety of creative solutions will be necessary in the future. NASA points out that pursuing these solutions is important because humankind cannot simply continue to live as it always has. It says, "Earth's climate has been relatively stable for the past 10,000 years, and this stability has allowed for the development of our modern civilization and agriculture. Our modern life is tailored to that stable climate and not the much warmer climate of the next thousand-plus years. As our climate changes, we will need to adapt."[89]

SOURCE NOTES

Introduction: Health and Climate Are Inseparable

1. US Environmental Protection Agency, "Climate Change and Human Health," February 27, 2023. www.epa.gov.
2. US Environmental Protection Agency, "Climate Change and Human Health."
3. Alexa K. Jay et al., "Ch. 1. Overview: Understanding Risks, Impacts, and Responses," *The Fifth National Climate Assessment*, 2023. https://nca2023.globalchange.gov.
4. World Health Organization, "Climate Change and Health," October 30, 2021. www.who.int.
5. Mary H. Hayden et al., "Ch. 15. Human Health," *The Fifth National Climate Assessment*, 2023. https://nca2023.globalchange.gov.
6. US Environmental Protection Agency, "Climate Equity," January 2, 2024. www.epa.gov.
7. Srilata Kammila, "The Climate Crisis Is a Health Crisis," June 7, 2022. www.undp.org.

Chapter One: Heat-Related Threats to Human Health

8. Samantha Chery and Terrence McCoy, "Woman Dies After Going to Sweltering Taylor Swift Concert in Rio," *Washington Post*, November 18, 2023. www.washingtonpost.com.
9. Quoted in *Marie Claire*, "Taylor Swift, the Exorbitant Heat of Rio de Janeiro and the Absolute Chaos: A Report on the 1st Concert of the Eras Tour in Brazil," November 18, 2023. https://revistamarieclaire.globo.com.
10. Quoted in Chery and McCoy, "Woman Dies After Going to Sweltering Taylor Swift Concert in Rio."
11. Roberto Delgado et al., "Ch. 2. Climate Trends," *The Fifth National Climate Assessment*, 2023. https://nca2023.globalchange.gov.
12. World Weather Attribution, "Extreme Heat in North America, Europe and China in July 2023 Made Much More Likely by Climate Change," July 25, 2023. www.worldweatherattribution.org.
13. Steven Woolf et al., "The Healthcare Costs of Extreme Heat," Center for American Progress, June 27, 2023. www.americanprogress.org.
14. Quoted in National Weather Service, "Real Life Stories from Excessive Heat Victims." www.weather.gov.
15. Quoted in National Weather Service, "Real Life Stories from Excessive Heat Victims."
16. Hayden et al., "Ch. 15. Human Health."

17. Ajit Niranjan, "Heatwave Last Summer Killed 61,000 People in Europe, Research Finds," *The Guardian* (Manchester, UK), July 10, 2023. www.theguardian.com.

18. Quoted in Niranjan, "Heatwave Last Summer Killed 61,000 People in Europe, Research Finds."

19. Jingwen Liu et al. "Heat Exposure and Cardiovascular Health Outcomes: A Systematic Review and Meta-analysis," *The Lancet Planetary Health*, June 2022. www.thelancet.com.

20. Quoted in Nouran Salahieh and Laura Studley, "Extreme Heat in Arizona Increased Hospitalizations to Pandemic Levels at One Medical Center," CNN, July 18, 2023. www.cnn.com.

21. Quoted in Salahieh and Studley, "Extreme Heat in Arizona Increased Hospitalizations to Pandemic Levels at One Medical Center."

22. Woolf et. al., "The Healthcare Costs of Extreme Heat."

23. Bonnie Schneider, *Taking the Heat: How Climate Change Is Affecting Your Mind, Body, and Spirit and What You Can Do About It.* New York: Simon Element, 2021, p. 51.

24. Huw Oliver, "How Paris Plans to Become Europe's Greenest City by 2030," TimeOut, November 2, 2021. www.timeout.com.

Chapter Two: How Changing Air Quality Impacts Health

25. American Lung Association, "State of the Air 2023: Key Findings," 2023. www.lung.org.

26. Quoted in Josie Garthwaite, "Stanford Researchers Find Wildfire Smoke Is Unraveling Decades of Air Quality Gains, Exposing Millions of Americans to Extreme Pollution Levels," Stanford News, September 22, 2022. https://news.stanford.edu.

27. Quoted in Sarah Gibbens and Amy McKeever, "How Wildfire Smoke Affects Your Body—and How You Can Protect Yourself," *National Geographic*, June 7, 2023. www.nationalgeographic.com.

28. Centers for Disease Control and Prevention, "Allergens and Pollen," August 21, 2020. www.cdc.gov.

29. American Lung Association, "State of the Air 2023."

30. World Health Organization, "Air Pollution: The Invisible Health Threat," July 12, 2023. www.who.int.

31. Laura López González, "Unmasking the Dangers: The Hidden Health Risks of Wildfire Smoke," University of California, San Francisco, August 15, 2023. www.ucsf.edu.

32. Quoted in Eva Frederick, "What We Don't Know About Wildfire Smoke Is Likely Hurting Us," *Science*, February 14, 2020. www.science.org.

33. Centers for Disease Control and Prevention, "Allergens and Pollen."

34. Theresa MacPhail, *Allergic: Our Irritated Bodies in a Changing World.* New York: Random House, 2023, p. xvii.

35. Quoted in Seth Borenstein and Melina Walling, "Climate Change Keeps Making Wildfires and Smoke Worse. Scientists Call It the 'New Normal,'" AP News, July 1, 2023. https://apnews.com.
36. Quoted in Erika Edwards, "Adults Are Getting Allergies for the First Time. Thanks, Climate Change," NBC News, April 25, 2023. www.nbcnews.com.
37. Quoted in Edwards, "Adults Are Getting Allergies for the First Time."
38. Jay et al., "Ch. 1. Overview."
39. Jack Foersterling, "Tackling Climate Change One Ride at a Time," PeopleForBikes, September 20, 2021. www.peopleforbikes.org.
40. Clean Air Fund, "Case Studies: Innovative Finance for Air Quality," 2023. www.cleanairfund.org.

Chapter Three: The Effects of Extreme Weather Events on Health

41. Kate Bartlett, "Cyclone Freddy Broke Records and Ravaged Countries. How Does the Healing Begin?," NPR, March 17, 2023. www.npr.org.
42. US Environmental Protection Agency, "Climate Change Indicators: Weather and Climate, July 26, 2023. www.epa.gov.
43. National Aeronautics and Space Administration, "Extreme Weather and Climate Change." https://climate.nasa.gov.
44. Quoted in William Brangham, "Climate Scientist Discusses This Summer's Extreme Weather and Long-Term Trends," PBS, September 6, 2023. www.pbs.org.
45. Quoted in Arvind Chhabra, "Himachal Pradesh: Shimla Residents Reel from Devastation Caused by Heavy Rains," BBC, August 28, 2023. www.bbc.com.
46. Quoted in Brangham, "Climate Scientist Discusses This Summer's Extreme Weather and Long-Term Trends."
47. Quoted in Brangham, "Climate Scientist Discusses This Summer's Extreme Weather and Long-Term Trends."
48. Centers for Disease Control and Preventions, "Precipitation Extremes: Heavy Rainfall, Flooding, and Droughts," December 21, 2020. www.cdc.gov.
49. Quoted in NJ Spotlight News, "As Floodwaters Receded, Poisonous Mold Flourished in NJ Homes," June 2, 2023. www.njspotlightnews.org.
50. American Psychiatric Association, "How Extreme Weather Events Affect Mental Health," 2023. www.psychiatry.org.
51. Quoted in Stephen Simpson et al., "For Many Central Texans, Latest Bout of Cold Weather and Outages Reopens Old Wounds," Texas Tribune, February 2, 2023. www.texastribune.org.
52. Quoted in Simpson et al., "For Many Central Texans, Latest Bout of Cold Weather and Outages Reopens Old Wounds."

53. US Environmental Protection Agency, "Iowa City, Iowa Closes Vulnerable Wastewater Facility," April 24, 2023. www.epa.gov.

54. Quoted in Katie Brigham, "What It Takes to Relocate a Town Facing Sea Level Rise," CNBC, August 22, 2023. www.cnbc.com.

55. Adi Renaldi, "Indonesia's Giant Capital City Is Sinking. Can the Government's Plan Save It?," *National Geographic*, August 1, 2022. www.nationalgeographic.co.uk.

Chapter Four: Vector-Borne Diseases and Human Health

56. Quoted in Stephanie Colombini, "In Florida's Local Malaria Outbreak, Forgotten Bite Led to Surprise Hospitalization," NPR, July 26, 2023. www.npr.org.

57. Centers for Disease Control and Prevention, "Climate Change Increases the Number and Geographic Range of Disease-Carrying Insects and Ticks." www.cdc.gov.

58. Camila Mora et al., Over Half of Known Human Pathogenic Diseases Can Be Aggravated by Climate Change," *Nature Climate Change*, August 8, 2022. www.nature.com.

59. Centers for Disease Control and Prevention, "A National Public Health Framework for the Prevention and Control of Vector-Borne Diseases in Humans, Atlanta, Georgia," September 2020. www.cdc.gov.

60. US Environmental Protection Agency, "Climate Change Indicators: Lyme Disease," November 1, 2023. www.epa.gov.

61. US Environmental Protection Agency, "Climate Change Indicators: Lyme Disease."

62. Quoted in Jeffrey Klugger, "How Climate Change Affects Ticks and Lyme Disease," *Time*, March 13, 2023. https://time.com.

63. Quoted in Pien Huang, "The Relationship Between Climate Change and Rising Disease," NPR, March 19, 2023. www.npr.org.

64. World Mosquito Program, "Explainer: How Climate Change Is Amplifying Mosquito-Borne Diseases." www.worldmosquitoprogram.org.

65. Felipe J. Colón-González et al., "Projecting the Risk of Mosquito-Borne Diseases in a Warmer and More Populated World: A Multimodel, Multi-scenario Intercomparison Modelling Study," *The Lancet Planetary Health*, July 2021. www.thelancet.com.

66. World Mosquito Program, " Explainer."

67. Laura Norris, "Is the Threat of Malaria Increasing?," Bill & Melinda Gates Foundation, October 2, 2023. www.gatesfoundation.org.

68. Georgie Darling, "A Moment That Changed Me: Dengue Fever Put Me in the Hospital—and Taught Me to Love My Body," *The Guardian* (Manchester, UK), March 23, 2022. www.theguardian.com.

69. Drugs for Neglected Diseases initiative, "Five Ways Innovation Is Changing the Fight Against Neglected Tropical Diseases," January 27, 2022. https://dndi.org.

70. Stephanie Nolen, "The Gamble: Can Genetically Modified Mosquitos End Disease?," *New York Times*, September 29, 2023. www.nytimes.com.

71. Quoted in Stephanie Nolen, "The Gamble."

Chapter Five: The Health Consequences of Changing Water Quality

72. United Nations, "Water and Climate Change." www.unwater.org.

73. Intergovernmental Panel on Climate Change, "Chapter 4: Water," 2022. www.ipcc.ch.

74. Quoted in OxFam International, "Drought in East Africa: 'If the Rains Do Not Come, None of Us Will Survive.'" www.oxfam.org.

75. Jay et al., "Ch. 1. Overview."

76. Quoted in Good Men Project, "What Is Seawater Intrusion? A Hydrogeologist Explains the Shifting Balance Between Fresh and Saltwater at the Coast," November 7, 2023. https://goodmenproject.com.

77. US Environmental Protection Agency, "Climate Adaptation and Harmful Algal Blooms," June 21, 2023. www.epa.gov.

78. Sandra Hoffmann et al., "Climate Change Projected to Increase Costs of U.S. Vibrio Infections," US Department of Agriculture Economic Research Service, June 26, 2023. https://www.ers.usda.gov.

79. Rebecca Lindsey, "Drought Parches the Central Amazon in October 2023," National Oceanic and Atmospheric Administration, October 30, 2023. www.climate.gov3.

80. Quoted in Bruno Kelly and Steven Grattan, "In Brazil's Amazon, Drought Affects Locals' Access to Food and Water," Reuters, September 28, 2023. www.reuters.com.

81. Quoted in Kelly and Grattan, "In Brazil's Amazon, Drought Affects Locals' Access to Food and Water."

82. Quoted in Denise Chow, "Three Islands Disappeared in the Past Year. Is Climate Change to Blame?," NBC News, June 9, 2019. www.nbcnews.com.

83. Quoted in ReliefWeb, "Kiribati: The Remote Island Nation Faces a Triple Threat to Health," May 16, 2023. https://reliefweb.int.

84. Carbon Almanac Network, *The Carbon Almanac*. New York: Penguin Random House, 2022, p. 119.

85. United Nations, "Water and Climate Change."

86. World Bank, "Rainwater Harvesting in Yemen: A Durable Solution for Water Scarcity," August 26, 2022. www.worldbank.org.

87. National Oceanic and Atmospheric Administration, "Understanding Living Shorelines." www.fisheries.noaa.gov.

88. Chesapeake Bay Foundation, "Successful Shorelines Require a Sea Change," September 15, 2022. www.cbf.org.

89. National Aeronautics and Space Administration, "Responding to Climate Change." https://climate.nasa.gov.

ORGANIZATIONS AND WEBSITES

Climate Change Impacts
www.epa.gov/climateimpacts
This website of the US Environmental Protection Agency is focused on the way climate change is affecting society and the ecosystem. It provides resources on air quality, water quality, and health.

Intergovernmental Panel on Climate Change
www.ipcc.ch
This international organization was created in 1988 and publishes regular assessments on the effects of climate change. Its website provides these reports in addition to resources about mitigation and adaptation options.

National Oceanic and Atmospheric Administration (NOAA)
www.noaa.gov
The NOAA is a government agency that provides weather information, storm warnings, and climate monitoring. Its website has many articles about climate change and human health, including predictions about the future. It also has links to climate information from the National Weather Service.

US Global Change Research Program
www.globalchange.gov
This federal agency works to understand how climate change will impact the planet and society. Its website contains many resources about how climate change is affecting human health, including reports, webinars, podcasts, and videos.

World Meteorological Organization
https://public.wmo.int
The World Meteorological Organization is an agency of the United Nations. Its website has links to articles, fact sheets, and videos about global weather patterns and the way they are affecting human health.

FOR FURTHER RESEARCH

Books

Carbon Almanac Network, *The Carbon Almanac*. New York: Penguin Random House, 2022.

Theresa MacPhail, *Allergic: Our Irritated Bodies in a Changing World*. New York: Random House, 2023.

Joseph J. Romm, *Climate Change: What Everyone Needs to Know*. New York: Oxford University Press, 2022.

Bonnie Schneider, *Taking the Heat: How Climate Change Is Affecting Your Mind, Body, and Spirit and What You Can Do About It*. New York: Simon Element, 2021.

Internet Sources

American Lung Association, "State of the Air 2023: Key Findings," 2023. www.lung.org.

Centers for Disease Control and Prevention, "Climate Effects on Health," April 25, 2022. www.cdc.gov.

Mary H. Hayden et al., "Ch. 15. Human Health," *The Fifth National Climate Assessment*, 2023. https://nca2023.globalchange.gov.

Dennis Lupenga, "Climate Stories: Meet the People Affected by Extreme Weather," WaterAid. www.wateraid.org.

US Environmental Protection Agency, "Climate Change and Human Health," February 27, 2023. www.epa.gov.

Steven Woolf et al., "The Healthcare Costs of Extreme Heat," Center for American Progress, June 27, 2023. www.americanprogress.org.

World Mosquito Program, "Explainer: How Climate Change Is Amplifying Mosquito-Borne Diseases." www.worldmosquitoprogram.org.

World Weather Attribution, "Extreme Heat in North America, Europe and China in July 2023 Made Much More Likely by Climate Change," July 25, 2023. www.worldweatherattribution.org.

PICTURE CREDITS

Cover: nechaevkon/Shutterstock.com

6: US Army Photo/Alamy Stock Photo

10: Fausto Maia/ZUMAPRESS/Newscom

13: New Africa/Shutterstock.com

15: MAXPPP/Alamy Stock Photo

18: PeopleImages.com - Yuri A/Shutterstock.com

23: lev radin/Shutterstock.com

24: connel/Shutterstock.com

27: Xinhua/Alamy Stock Photo

29: dpa picture alliance/Alamy Stock Photo

33: Kevin Herbian/ZUMAPRESS/Newscom

36: Eye Ubiquitous/Alamy Stock Photo

39: Phil Degginger/Alamy Stock Photo

43: Helmut Fricke/dpa/picture-alliance/Newscom

46: Eye Ubiquitous/Alamy Stock Photo

48: Cavan Images/Alamy Stock Photo

52: Cecile Marion/Alamy Stock Photo